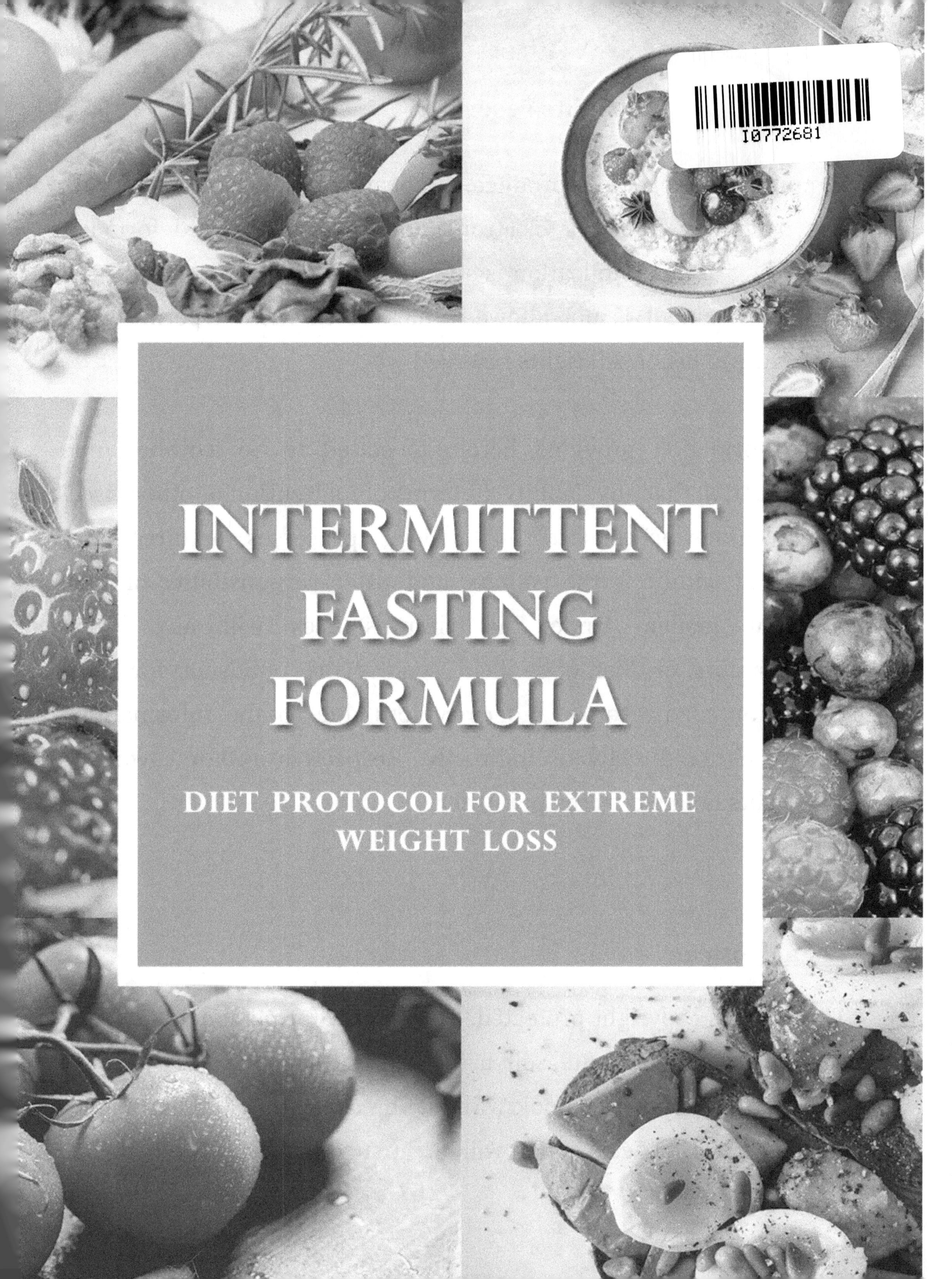
INTERMITTENT FASTING FORMULA
DIET PROTOCOL FOR EXTREME WEIGHT LOSS

Disclaimer Notice:

Please note the information contained within this document is for educational and entertainment purposes only. Every attempt has been made to provide accurate, up to date and reliable complete information. No warranties of any kind are expressed or implied. Readers acknowledge that the author is not engaging in the rendering of legal, financial, medical or professional advice.

By reading this document, the reader agrees that under no circumstances are we responsible for any losses, direct or indirect, which are incurred as a result of the use of information contained within this document, including, but not limited to, —errors, omissions, or inaccuracies.

TABLE OF CONTENTS

Conclusion **81**

Introduction

Why is Intermittent Fasting so Popular?

Obesity is becoming an increasing problem. So, it's no wonder that so many people are looking for a better way to lose weight. Traditional diets that restrict calories often fail to work for many people. It's difficult to follow this type of diet in the long-term. This often leads to yo-yo dieting – an endless cycle of weight loss and gain. Not only does this often result in mental health issues, it can also lead to even more weight gain overall.

It comes as no surprise, then, that many people have been searching for a diet that can be maintained long-term. Intermittent fasting is one such diet. More of a lifestyle change than an eating plan, it is different from regular diets. Many followers of intermittent fasting find it easy to follow for extended periods. Even better, it helps them to lose weight effectively.

However, this type of eating plan also offers benefits beyond weight loss. Many people believe that it can offer other health and wellness benefits too. Some of those benefits are even said to stretch further – some say it makes them more productive and focused. As a result, they can become more successful in the workplace. There have been recent stories in the media of CEOs who claim their success is all down to intermittent fasting.

Yet, the benefits don't stop there. There is some evidence to show that intermittent fasting (or IF) helps wellness in other ways too. It has been said to improve blood sugar levels and immunity. It may boost brain function, decrease inflammation and repair cells in the body too.

With all of this in mind, it's easy to see why this way of eating is becoming more popular. Here, we'll take a closer look at why intermittent fasting works to promote weight loss. We'll examine the benefits of this lifestyle change and we'll show you how to get started with this diet protocol.

CHAPTER 1

WHAT IS INTERMITTENT FASTING?

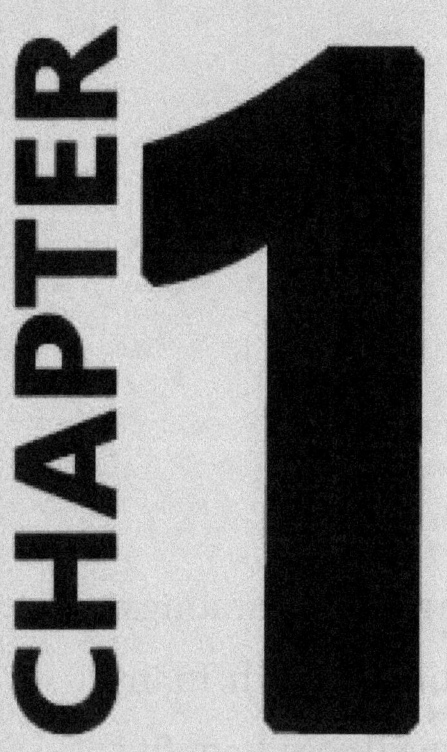

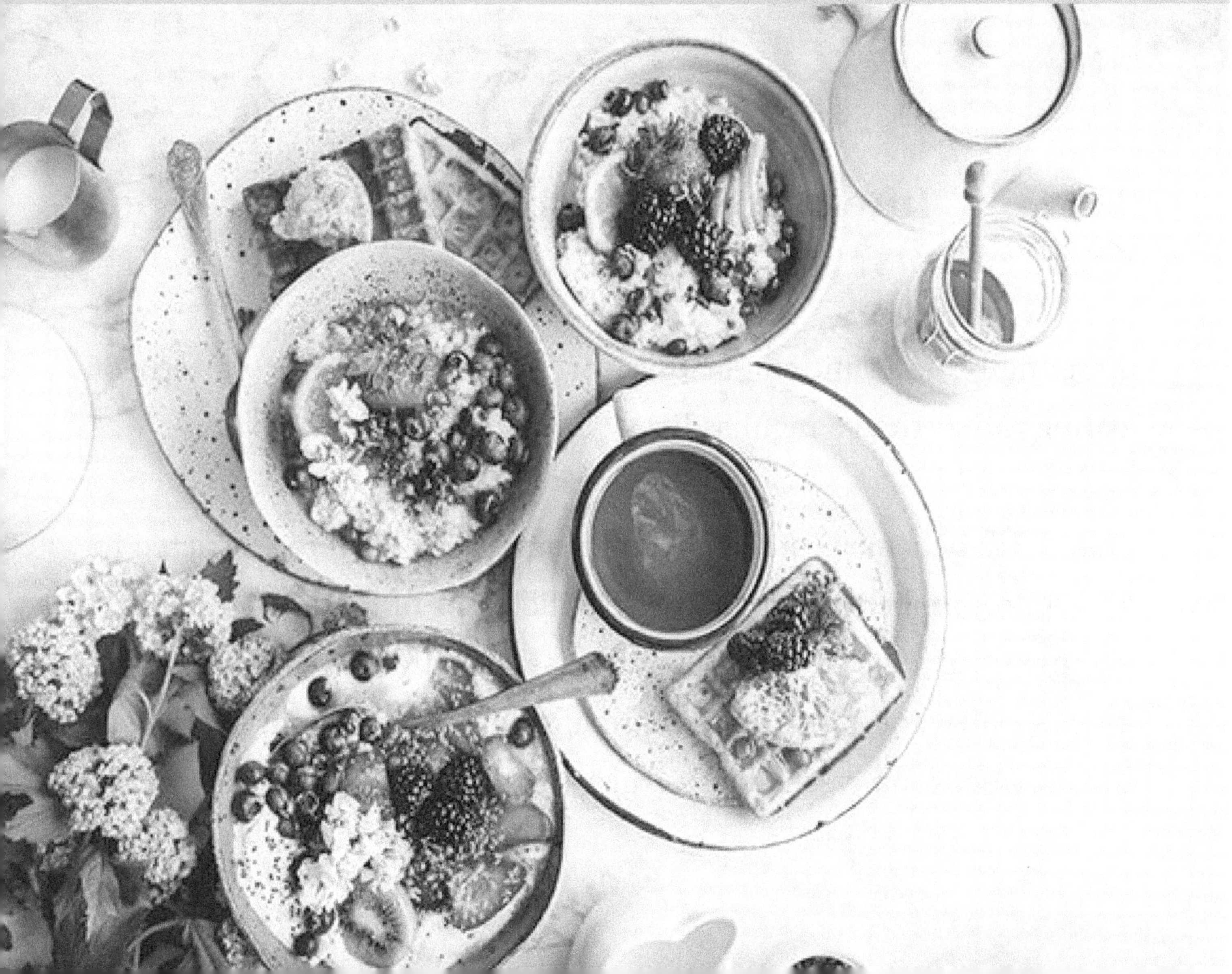

Chapter 1 – What is Intermittent Fasting?

Intermittent fasting is rapidly becoming a popular choice amongst those trying to lose weight. However, it's also popular with many other people too who want to reap its health and wellness benefits. So, what is intermittent fasting all about?

How is Intermittent Fasting Different from Other Diets?

Essentially, intermittent fasting (or IF for short) is a pattern of eating rather than a regular diet.

Standard diets focus on what you're eating. Dieters are restricted to a certain number of calories or specific types of food. This leads to dieters thinking constantly about what they are and aren't allowed to eat. Fatty and sugary foods are absolutely forbidden. There is a strong focus on vegetables, fruit and low-fat, low-sugar meals.

Those following these ways of eating often end up fantasizing about treats and snacks. While they may lose weight, they may struggle to stick to their eating plan in the long-term.

Intermittent fasting is different. It is a lifestyle rather than a diet. It involves eating patterns during which you cycle between windows of fasting and eating. Unlike other diets, it doesn't focus on what you're eating. Instead, it focuses on when you should eat. Some dieters enjoy the greater freedom this gives them. They can eat the foods they enjoy without guilt. Many people also find that it fits better into their lifestyles. However, there are some potential pitfalls when it comes to IF for weight loss.

The Origins of Intermittent Fasting

Intermittent fasting as a lifestyle choice is relatively new. However, the concept of fasting certainly isn't. There are verses in the Bible and Koran about fasting for religious purposes. Many religious people still fast today for religious reasons. The month of Ramadan remains a time when Muslims refrain from eating from sun-up to sun-down. Therefore, it's easy to see where the idea of intermittent fasting originates.

Even during ancient Greek civilizations, fasting was practiced. In many primitive cultures, fasting was part of many rituals. It has also formed the basis of political protests – for example by the suffragettes during the early 20th century.

Therapeutic fasting became a trend during the 1800s as a way of preventing or treating poor health. Carried out under a doctor's supervision, this type of fasting was adopted to treat many conditions from hypertension to headaches. Each fast was tailored to the individual's needs. It could be just a day or up to three months.

Although fasting fell out of favor as new medications were developed, it has recently re-emerged. In 2019, "intermittent fasting" was one of the most commonly searched terms. So, what should you know about it?

The Most Popular Types of Intermittent Fasting

There are plenty of different kinds of intermittent fasting. Each one has its own following. All follow the same principle of restricting food intake for a certain period of time. However, the length of the time and the gap between eating windows varies.

Perhaps the most popular IF method is the 16:8 fast. This involves an eating window of 8 hours followed by 16 hours of fasting. Many people find this the most convenient option for them. If they skip breakfast or dinner, they can fit it easily into their lifestyle.

Another popular IF option is the 24-hour fast. This is sometimes known as the Eat-Stop-Eat method. It involves eating normally one day then avoiding food for the following 24 hours. The gaps in between fasts could be as short as 24 hours or up to 72 hours.

The 5:2 fasting method is also popular. This involves eating normally for five days of the week. The other two consecutive days, the dieter should restrict their calorie consumption to around 500-600 calories.

Some IF dieters choose the 20:4 method. This involves concentrating all eating each day into a four-hour window. During the other 20 hours of the day, the dieter should eat no calories.

There are several other types of fasting diet. Some people follow extended fasts of up to 48 or 36 hours. Others fast for even more extended periods. If you're considering trying IF, you'll need to choose the right method for you.

Why do People Prefer Intermittent Fasting?

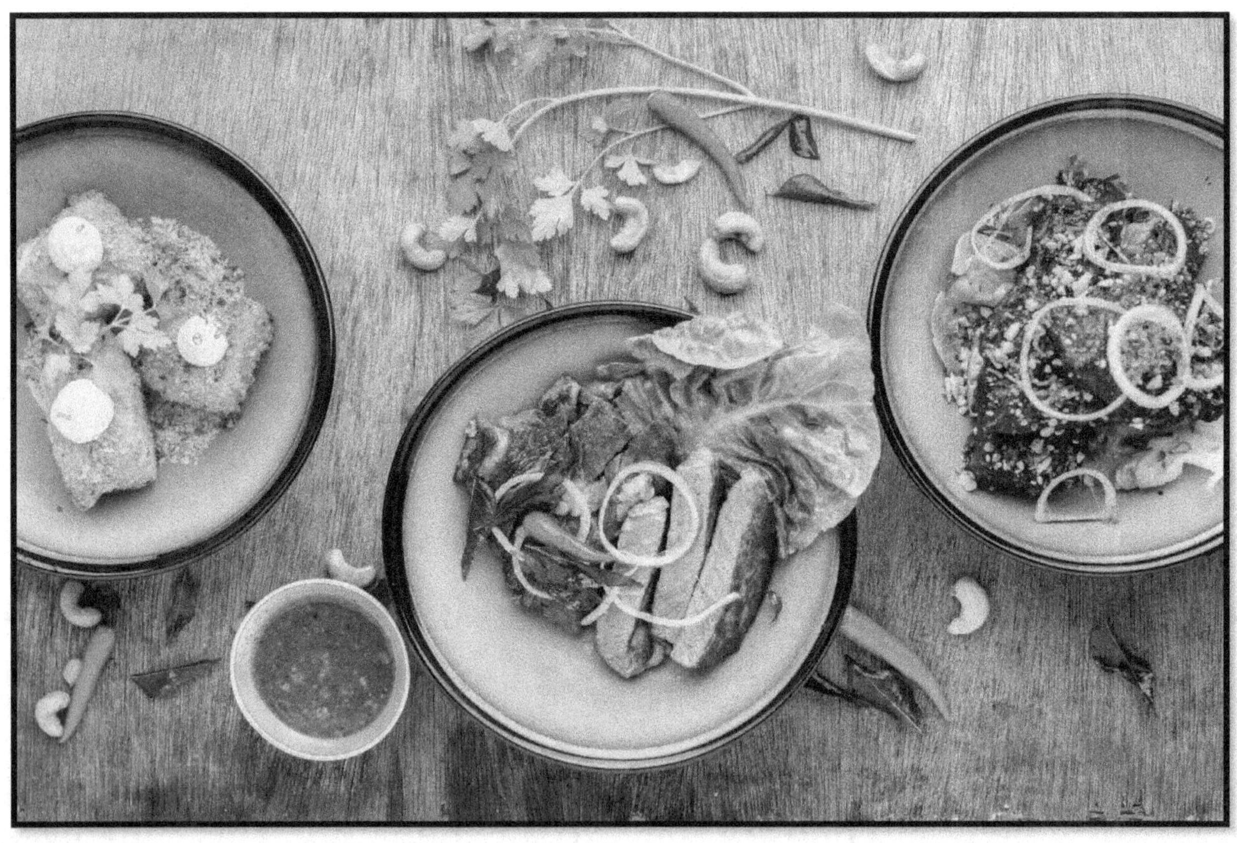

Unlike other types of dieting, IF allows dieters to eat pretty much what they want. They can eat the sugary or fatty foods they crave. They can go out to eat and not worry about calorie counting. They don't have to eat foods they don't enjoy. They don't have to feel as if they're depriving themselves of the things they love. It's easy to see why it's such a popular choice.

Not only that, but intermittent fasting offers many more benefits than other types of diet. Yes, it promotes rapid weight loss. However, it also helps dieters to feel more focused and be more productive. It helps them to feel healthier and more energetic. With the wellness benefits that this way of eating brings, it's no wonder people prefer it to regular diets.

CHAPTER 2

THE BENEFITS OF INTERMITTENT FASTING

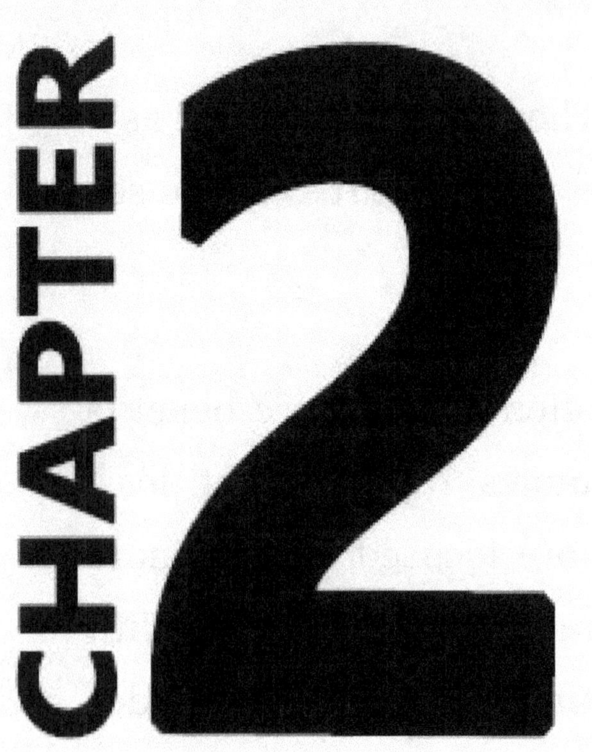

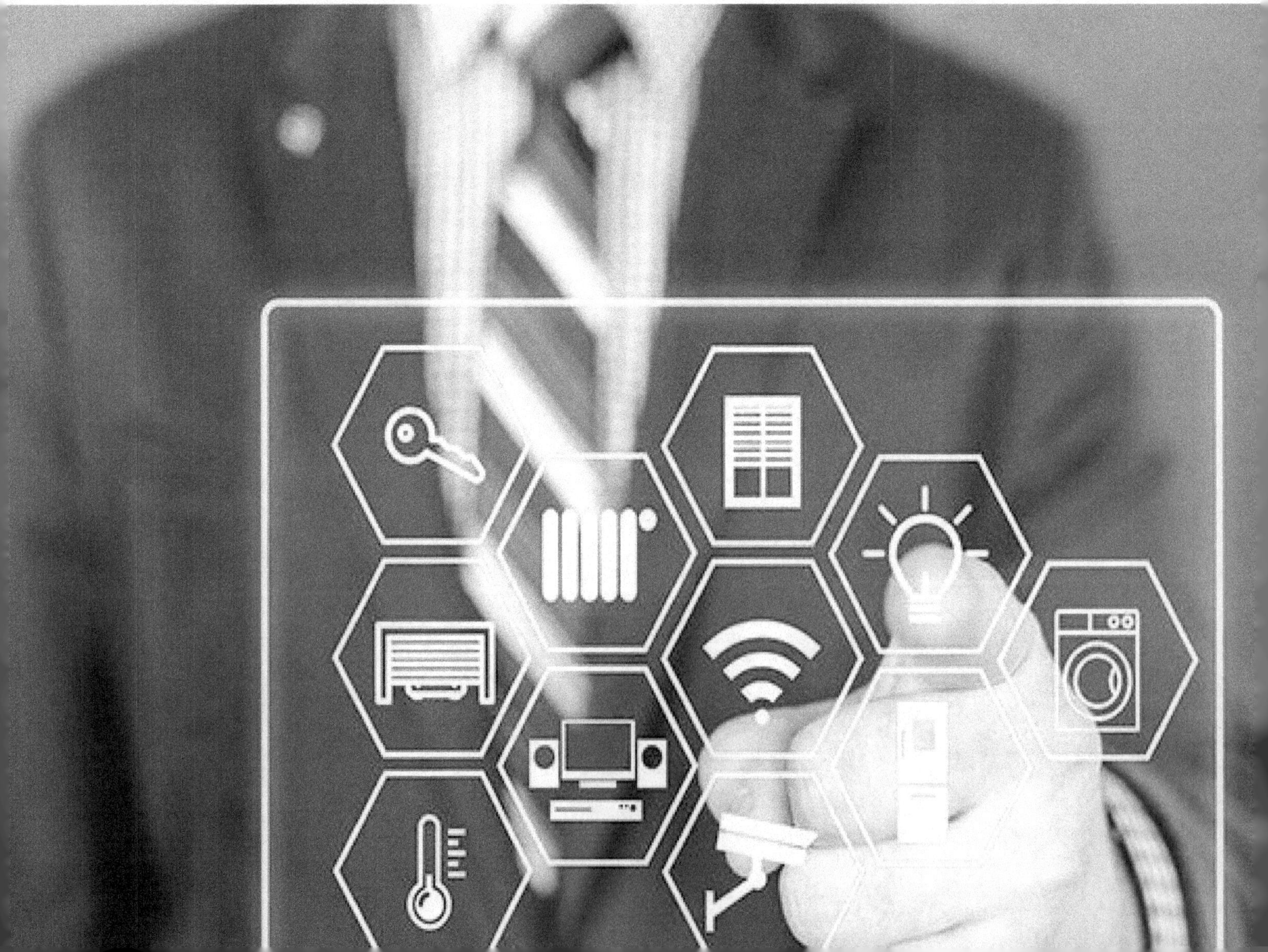

Chapter 2 – The Benefits of Intermittent Fasting

There are several benefits that those who follow an intermittent fasting lifestyle report. Here, we take a closer look at some of the most common.

Weight Loss

Many people who do intermittent fasting do so to lose weight rapidly. There is evidence to show that this way of eating helps you to shed the pounds more quickly. There are several reasons why IF helps weight loss. It enhances the function of the metabolism for faster fat burning.

It also reduces the number of calories you consume in 24 hours. By lowering insulin levels, increasing growth hormone levels and increasing norepinephrine, IF speeds up the breakdown of fat. It also facilitates the use of fat to produce energy.

Fasting for short periods of time has been shown to increase metabolic rate by up to 14 percent. This means you'll burn more calories. As a result, IF can help cause weight loss of up to 8 percent over a period of 3 – 24 weeks. That's an impressive loss!

Those who try IF report a reduction of 7 percent in the circumference of their waist. This indicates a loss of belly fat – the most harmful type of fat that results in disease.

As an added bonus, IF causes reduced muscle loss when compared to calorie restriction diets.

Repairing Cells

When you fast, your body's cells begin a process of removing waste cells. This is known as "autophagy". Autophagy involves the body's cells being broken down. It also involves the metabolization of dysfunctional and broken proteins that have built up over time in the cells.

What is the benefit of autophagy? Well, experts believe that it offers protection from the development of several diseases. These include Alzheimer's Disease and cancer.

Therefore, if you follow an intermittent fasting regime, you may help to protect yourself from diseases. As a result, you may live a longer and healthier life.

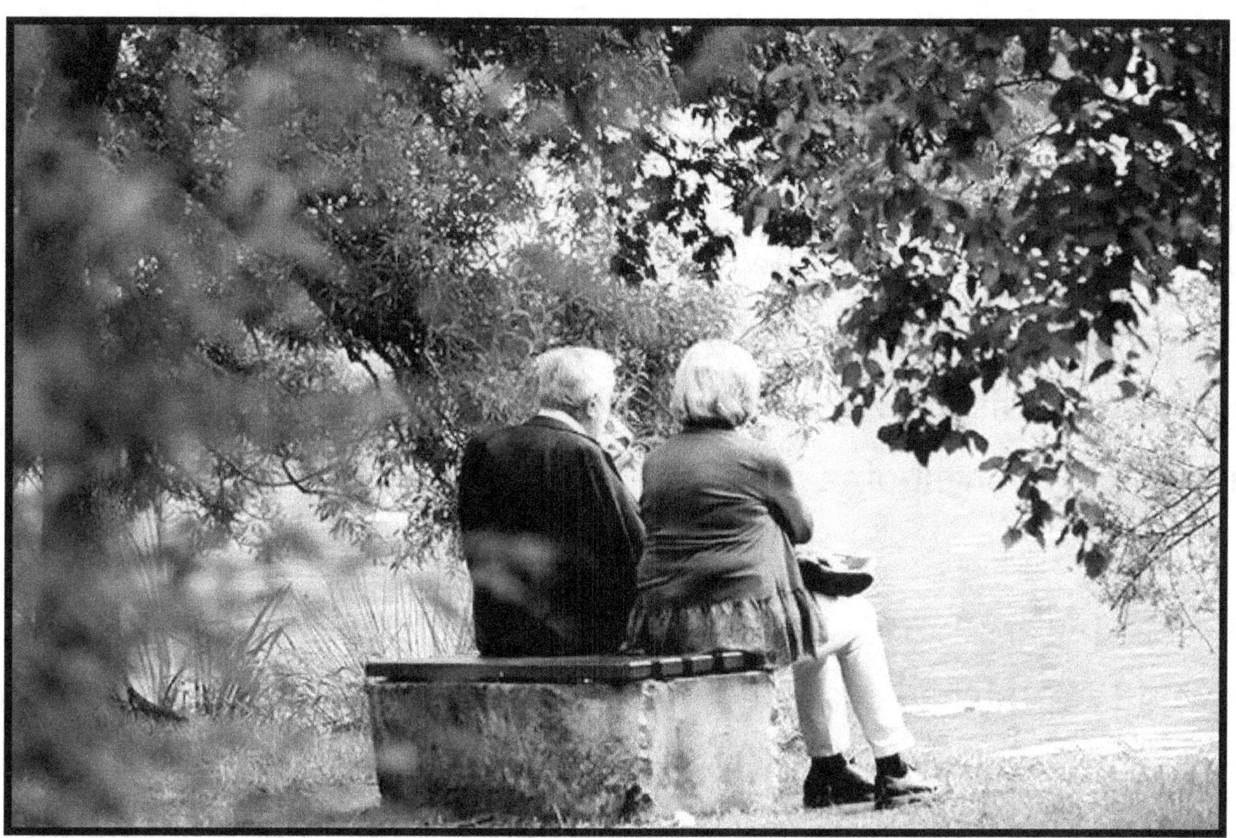

Insulin Sensitivity

More people than ever before have type 2 diabetes. The disease is becoming more common due to increasing obesity. The primary feature of diabetes is increased levels of sugar in the blood due to insulin resistance. If you can reduce insulin, your blood sugar level should decrease. This will offer excellent protection from developing type 2 diabetes.

Intermittent fasting has been proven to have a major benefit when it comes to insulin resistance. It can reduce blood sugar levels by an impressive amount. In studies into intermittent fasting with human participants, blood sugar levels decreased by up to 6 percent while fasting. As a result, fasting insulin levels can reduce by as much as 31 percent. This shows that IF could offer the benefit of reducing the chance of developing diabetes.

Another piece of research carried out amongst diabetic lab rats showed IF protected against damage to the kidneys. This is a severe complication associated with diabetes. So, again, it suggests that intermittent fasting is also a great option for anyone who already has diabetes.

Enhanced Brain Function

When something is good for your body, it's often good for your brain too. Intermittent fasting is known to improve several metabolic features. These are vital for good brain health.

Intermittent fasting has been shown to reduce oxidative stress. It also reduces inflammation and reduces the levels of sugar in the blood. Not only that, it reduces insulin resistance as we showed above. These are all key factors in enhancing brain function.

Studies that have taken place with lab rats have also shown that IF can help boost new nerve cell growth. This too offers benefits when it comes to brain function. Meanwhile, it also increases the level of BDNF (brain-derived neurotrophic factor). This is a brain hormone, and if you are deficient in it you may suffer from brain problems and depression. When you try intermittent fasting you will have better protection from these problems.

As an added advantage, studies in animals have shown that IF can protect against damage to the brain from strokes.

All of this suggests that intermittent fasting offers many brain health benefits.

Decreased Inflammation

It is known that oxidative stress is a key factor in chronic diseases as well as aging. Oxidative stress involves free radicals which are unstable molecules reacting with other key molecules such as DNA and protein. The result is damage to those molecules that causes harm in the body.

There have been several studies to prove that IF can help improve your body's ability to resist oxidative stress. Other studies have also shown it can help to combat inflammation which also drives many common diseases.

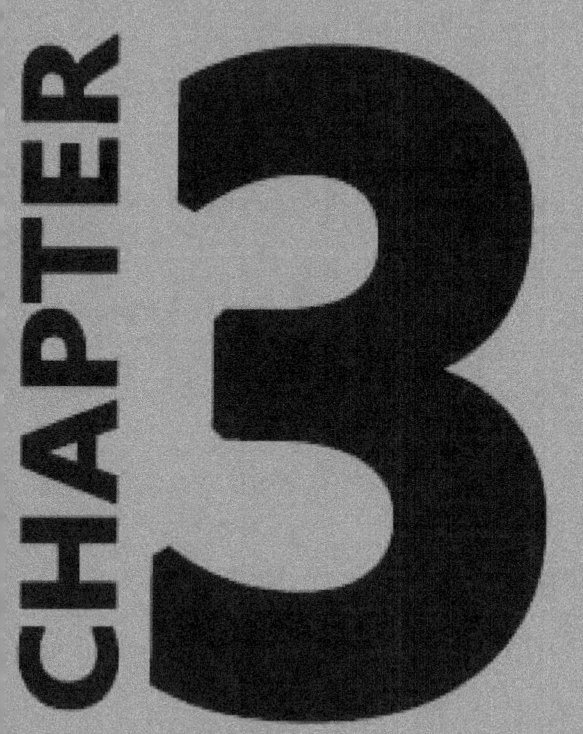

3

WHY DOES
INTERMITTENT FASTING
HELP TO PROMOTE
WEIGHT LOSS?

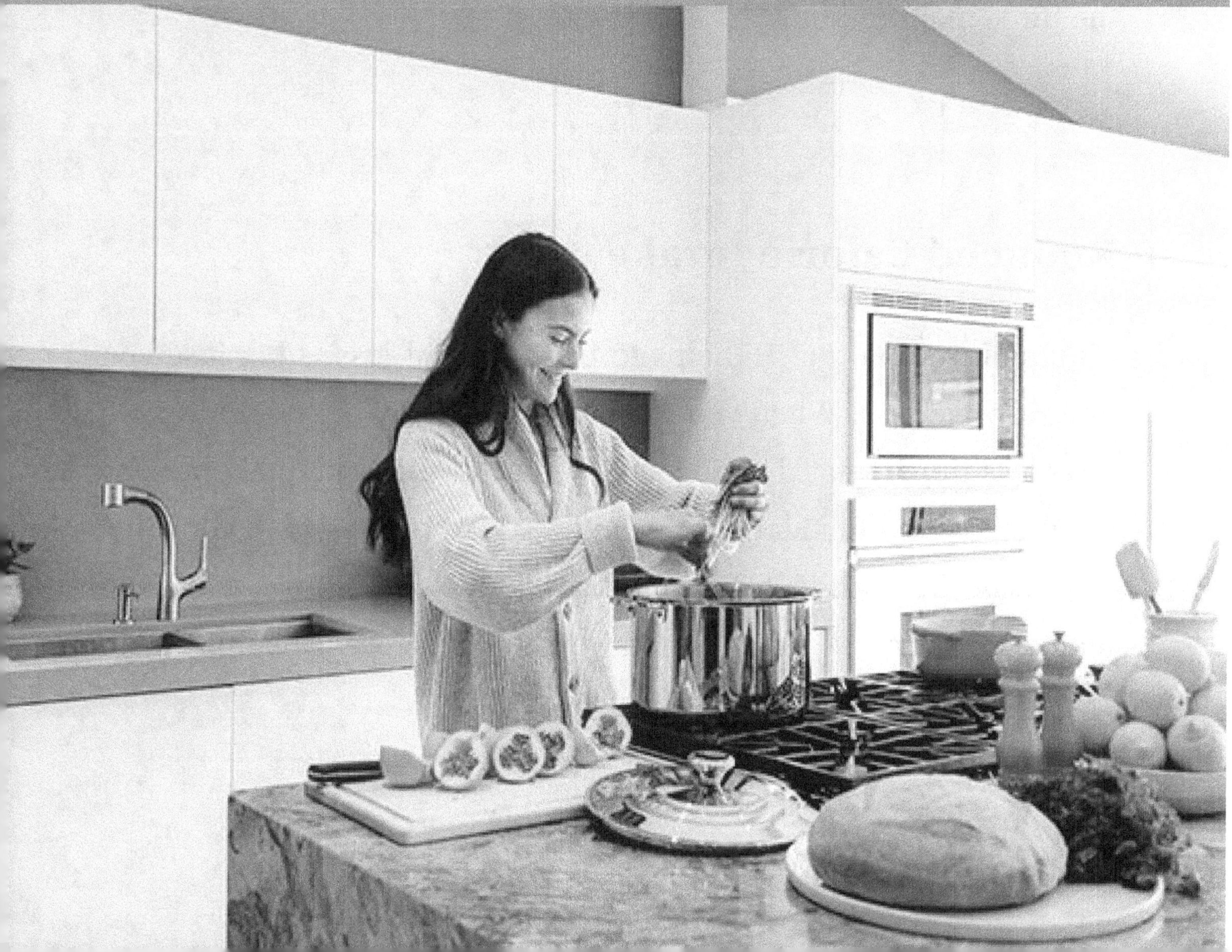

Chapter 3 – Why Does Intermittent Fasting Help to Promote Weight Loss?

Although intermittent fasting offers many benefits, the greatest one is weight loss. Most people who embark on this lifestyle are hoping to shed pounds and maintain a healthy bodyweight. So, why does intermittent fasting help to promote weight loss? Here, we look at the three main reasons.

Reduced Calorie Intake

The main reason that IF helps to boost weight loss is because you naturally eat less. When you only have a short eating window, you have less time to eat. Usually, you'll miss at least one meal per day in order to accommodate this schedule. As a result, you'll consume fewer calories within each 24-hour period. As you know, you must maintain a calorie deficit to shed weight. Therefore, IF helps you to reach your weight loss goals effectively.

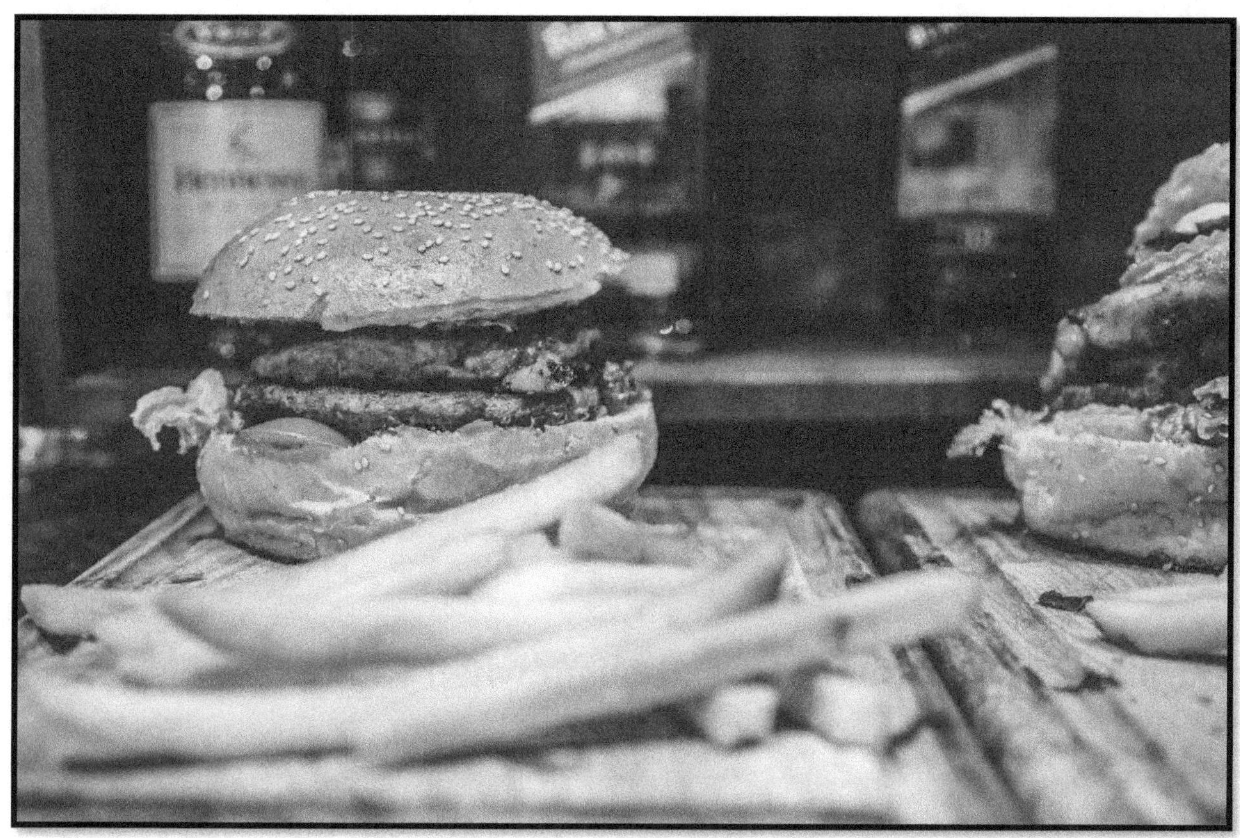

It's important to note, though, that some people fail to lose weight when they fast intermittently. This is because they don't reduce their calorie intake. During their eating window, they continue to eat as much as they would have if they had been eating normally. Therefore, they don't have the necessary calorie deficit to shed the pounds.

As long as you don't eat excessively during your eating window, you'll automatically reduce your calorie intake.

Hormonal Changes Boost Metabolism

The human body stores energy in the form of calories in body fat. If you don't eat, your body changes a number of things so that stored energy can be more accessible. These changes involve the activity of your nervous system. They also include major changes in a number of key hormones.

These changes occur in the metabolism when you're fasting:

- Insulin increases every time you eat. If you fast, your insulin level will dramatically decrease. A lower insulin level facilitates fat burning.

- HGH (Human Growth Hormone) skyrockets when you fast. It can increase by as much as five times its normal level. Growth hormone aids muscle gain and fat loss.

- Noradrenaline (Norepinephrine) is sent by the nervous system to your fat cells. This causes them to break down your body fat. It is turned into free fatty acids. These are then burned to produce energy.

Many people believe that if you fast your metabolism slows down. However, evidence shows that fasting in the short-term may boost fat burning. There have been two studies that have shown fasting for 48 hours increases metabolism up to 14 percent.

Reduced Insulin Levels Speed Fat Burning

You probably already know about insulin because of its importance for diabetics. People who have diabetes have to take insulin to maintain normal function. However, many people are unsure of what insulin does in the body or even what it is.

Insulin is a hormone that is made by your pancreas. Its job is to convert sugar (glucose) in the blood into energy. The cells then use that energy as fuel. Insulin also has another role to play in the body. It drives the storage of fat.

The level of insulin in the body will increase whenever you eat. It also decreases whenever you fast. The lower level of insulin caused when you fast can help to prevent excess storage of fat. It also helps

4

the body to mobilize the fat that is already stored. As a result, it can boost your fat and help you lose weight more rapidly.

IS INTERMITTENT FASTING SAFE?

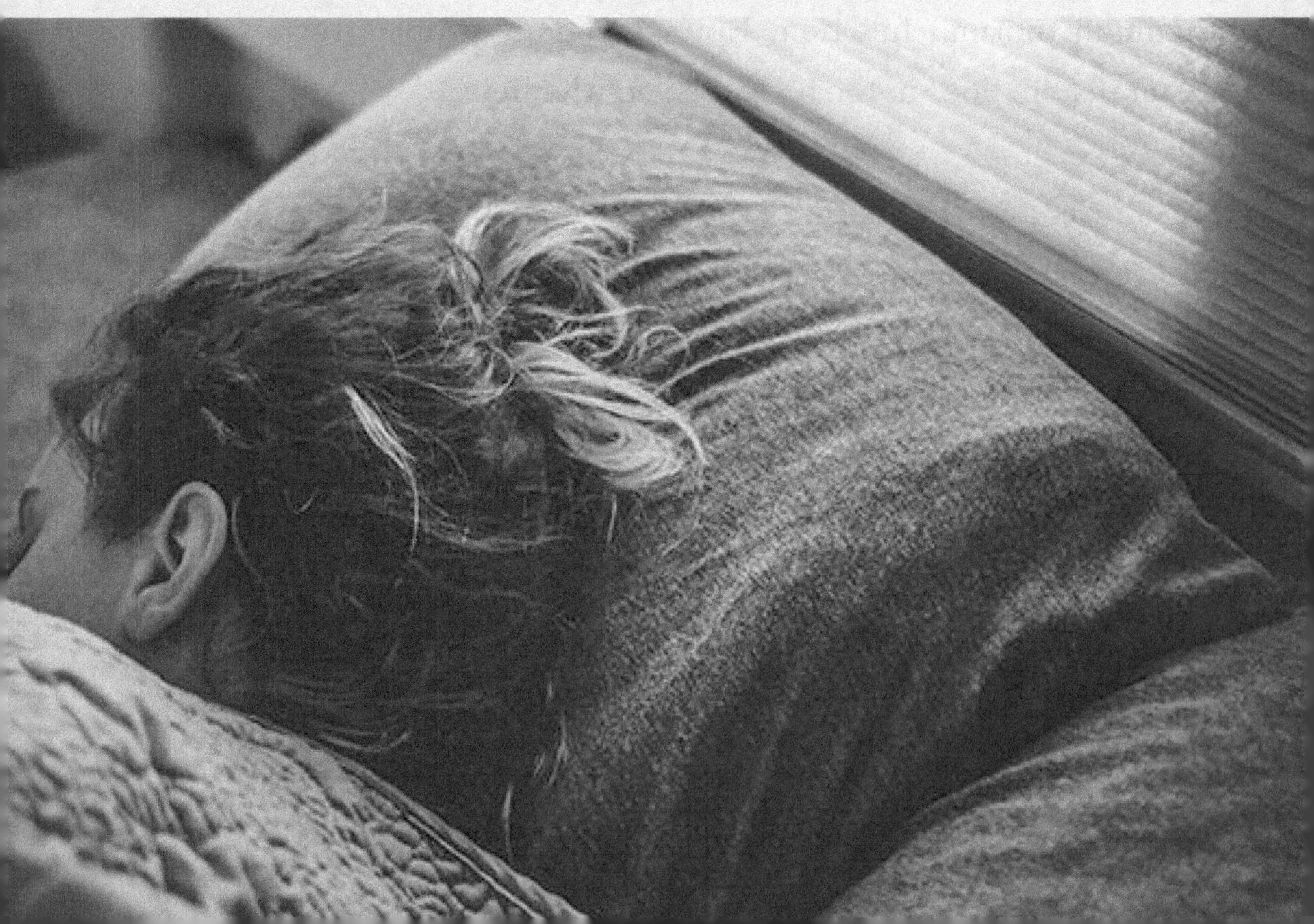

Chapter 4 – Is Intermittent Fasting Safe?

You may be keen to embark on an intermittent fasting lifestyle, but you might be concerned about safety. After all, not every diet is suitable for everyone.

A key factor in safe and successful weight loss is getting sufficient nutrition. If you don't get enough minerals, vitamins and protein, you could become ill. With too few calories and too restrictive an eating pattern, you may be unable to get enough nutrients. This may cause you to have medical issues.

The good news is that intermittent fasting appears to be a safe way of eating for most people. However, there are a few cases in which intermittent fasting should be avoided.

Who Should Avoid Intermittent Fasting?

There are a few groups of people who should take care when they do intermittent fasting. Although they may not need to avoid this lifestyle completely, they will need to show caution.

The first is children. Children are growing and developing. They therefore need to eat enough calories every day. They also need to get enough nutrients in the form of minerals and vitamins. Without enough protein they cannot grow properly. This could lead to a host of problems. Illnesses like scurvy can be caused due to lack of vitamins. Although some experts suggest that children can fast safely, it's something that should be approached with caution.

Diabetics should also take care when they do intermittent fasting. It's true to say that IF has a number of potential benefits for diabetics. This is because of the effect on insulin and blood sugar levels. However, there are some possible dangers. If you fast and have diabetes, your blood sugar level could drop dangerously low. This is especially likely if you're taking medication to control the condition.

When you don't eat, your blood sugar level will be lower. Your medication could then drop it even further leading to hypoglycemia. This can make you pass out, feel shaky or go into a coma. Another problem is that your blood sugar level may get too high when you do eat. This could happen if you consume too many carbohydrates.

If you're diabetic, always talk to a health professional before embarking on IF. You will also need to be more aware of the symptoms of low blood sugar. As long as you're cautious about what you eat and avoid hard exercise you may be fine.

The third and fourth groups who may wish to avoid IF are pregnant and breastfeeding women. Doctors usually recommend that these groups don't try intermittent fasting. This is because nutrition is absolutely vital at these stages in a woman's life. Not only is she feeding herself, she's feeding her baby. Therefore, she needs to consume sufficient calories and nutrients to support two people. This can be difficult when fasting intermittently. It should therefore only be attempted under medical supervision.

Could Intermittent Fasting Trigger an Eating Disorder?

For most people, intermittent fasting is a successful way of eating that causes no problems. However, there are some people who won't thrive on this lifestyle. Some people have a natural tendency to develop disordered eating behaviors. These people may need to avoid intermittent fasting if it triggers an eating disorder.

It's therefore vital to recognize if intermittent fasting has strayed into patterns of disordered eating. There are several symptoms to look for:

- You have anxiety about eating and food.
- You're feeling extremely fatigued.
- You're experiencing mood swings, menstrual changes and problems sleeping.

For those who have a genetic predisposition to disordered eating patterns, intermittent fasting can be dangerous. This is because there is a focus on not eating. Most diets focus on lowering your calorie intake by eating low calorie foods. IF minimizes your calorie intake by avoiding eating during certain periods. This can lead you to ignore the hunger signals of your body. Also, for someone with a tendency to develop eating disorders, you may become afraid of food due to IF. This is because you may start to associate avoiding food with losing weight. Your brain may begin to reward you for not eating and develop a fear of mealtimes.

Some people find that IF dieting causes them to binge eat. When they are in their eating window they end up over-indulging on high calorie foods. This mimics eating disorder behaviors. It's therefore important to be highly aware of any possible signs that your fasting is turning into an eating disorder.

What are the Side Effects of Intermittent Fasting?

Intermittent fasting offers many benefits but it has side effects too. These may affect each individual differently. Some of the effects you might experience include:

- Feeling grumpy, irritable and grouchy due to hunger
- Experiencing brain fog or excessive fatigue

- Obsessing about how much you can eat or what you can eat
- Persistent dizziness, headaches or nausea due to low blood sugar
- Hair loss due to a lack of nutrients
- Menstrual cycle changes due to rapid weight loss
- Constipation due to a lack of fiber, protein, vitamins or fluid
- The potential for developing an eating disorder
- Sleep disturbances

Most people won't experience these side effects to any serious extent. They will also usually disappear after a while. However, for some people, these problems are severe or long-lasting. If so, you may want to stop intermittent fasting until you seek medical advice.

Can Athletes try Intermittent Fasting?

Some athletes swear by intermittent fasting as a way to improve their athletic performance. However, there is mixed research on the subject. Some evidence suggests that if you don't consume enough carbohydrates, the duration and intensity of your training will suffer. Meanwhile, other research suggests that IF offers benefits for athletes.

Some of the potential benefits include:

- Growth hormone increases due to IF. This helps to boost muscle, cartilage and bone growth. It also improves your immune function – all good for athletes.
- It improves your metabolic flexibility so you can adapt more easily between energy sources. Your body will be better able to use carbs or fat as a source of fuel. It will also allow you to burn fat for much longer before your body switches to carbs. As a result, your insulin will stay low and your post-exercise recovery will improve.
- IF reduces inflammation. This aids your post-exercise recovery. When you exercise, you incur a large amount of inflammation that you must recover from. However, the faster that inflammation subsides the better. IF can speed the process up.

There are a few concerns, though. These include:

- It could cause a testosterone drop that is problematic because it impacts on muscle protein synthesis.
- You may find it difficult to eat sufficient calories to allow you to gain muscle.

Is it Safe for Women to Fast?

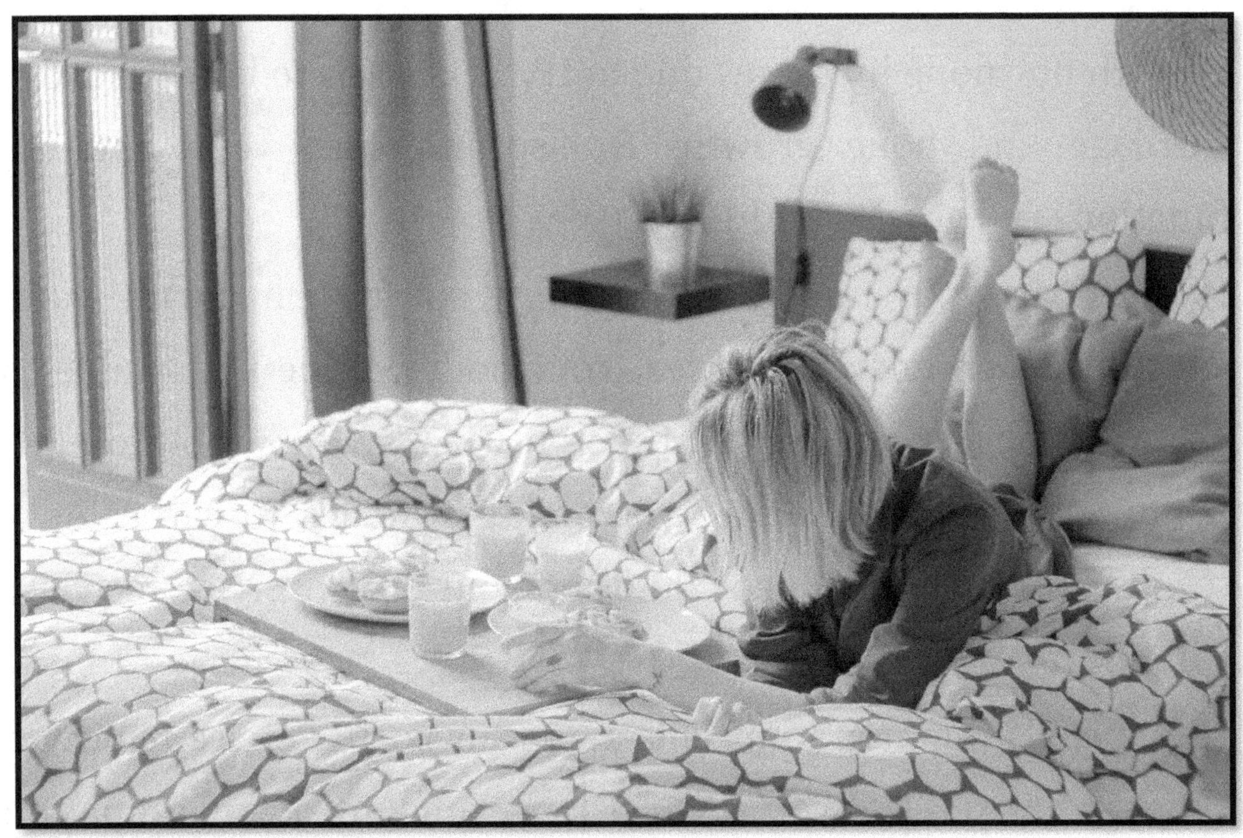

Many experts say that it's perfectly safe for women to fast. However, there is evidence that women have a greater sensitivity to starvation signals. When the body senses starvation, it increases production of ghrelin and leptin, the hunger hormones. This causes a negative energy balance and, often, wild mood swings as a result.

Women are also more prone to other hormonal imbalances if they do IF. This can cause menstrual cycle difficulties. It may also interfere with the production of the thyroid hormone. This could be problematic for anyone suffering from autoimmune conditions.

That doesn't mean, though, that women can't try intermittent fasting. It only means that they need to take more care. It may be better for women to begin with a gentler form of IF. Rather than a long fast, a 12-14 hour fast may be the best option.

Some women thrive on intermittent fasting while others find it doesn't suit them at all. It's worth experimenting to see if it works for you.

CHAPTER 5

A PROTOCOL FOR 16:8 INTERMITTENT FASTING

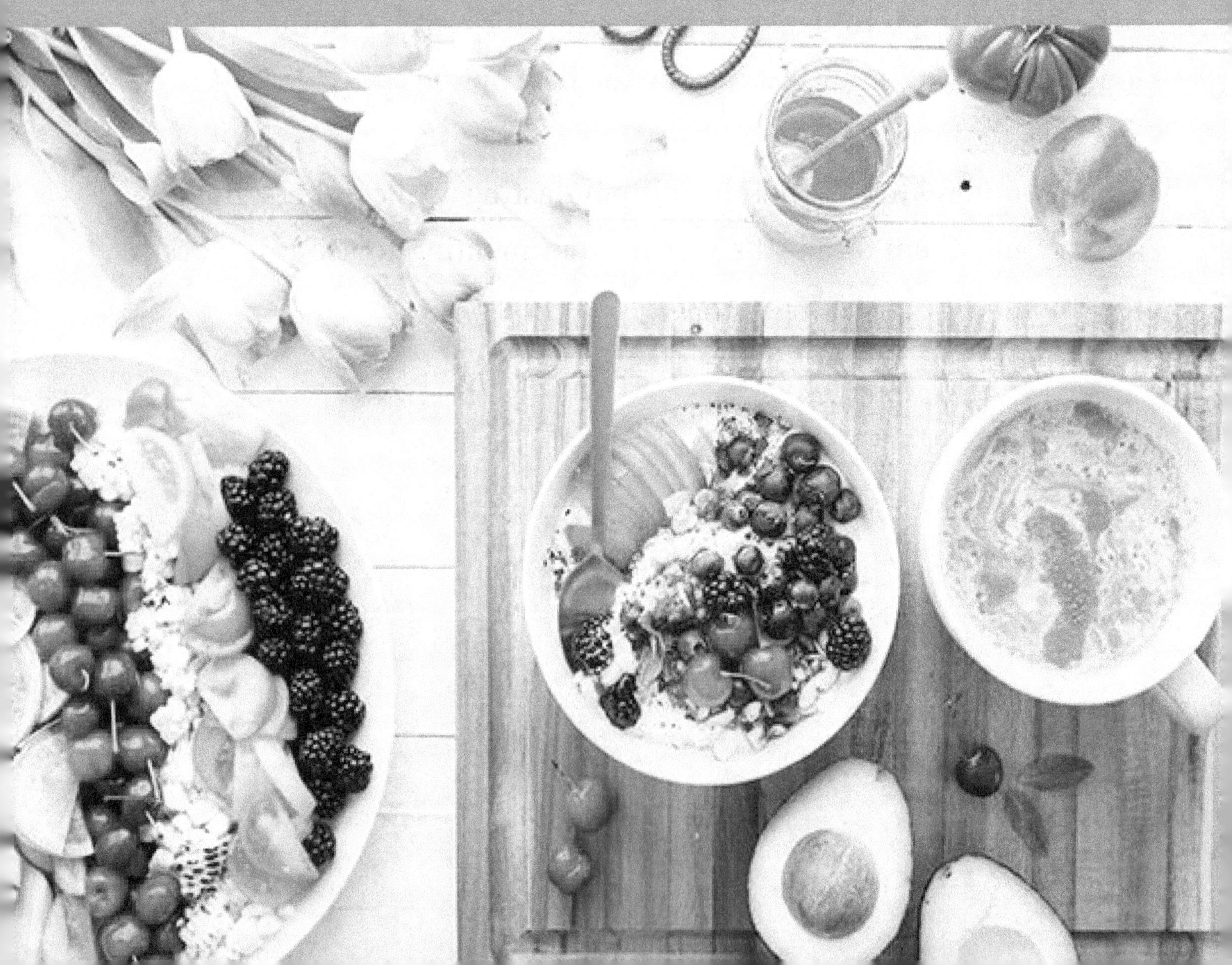

Chapter 5 – A Protocol for 16:8 Intermittent Fasting

If you're keen to try intermittent fasting, you may want to start with 16:8 fasting. This method involves fasting for 16 hours and then having an eating window of 8 hours. It is one of the most popular forms of this way of eating. If you're ready to get started, here is a protocol for 16:8 IF.

Choosing an Eating Window

When you're ready to begin 16:8 fasting, the first thing to do is choose an eating window. This 8-hour period can be at any time of the day. Therefore, you can choose the right time to suit your preferences and lifestyle. When you have chosen your preferred eight hours, you must limit your consumption of food to those hours.

How do you choose the right hours for you? Lots of people like an eating window of noon to 8 p.m. This is because they can fast overnight, skip breakfast and then enjoy lunch and dinner at the usual times. They can even add in a couple of healthy snacks into their regime.

For people who would prefer to have three meals a day, a 9 a.m. – 5 p.m. eating window may be best. This allows for breakfast at 9 a.m., lunch at noon then an early dinner at 4 p.m.

Others prefer to wait until early afternoon to break their fast then to have their last meal later before bed.

Whichever eating window you choose, make sure it's one that fits with your lifestyle patterns. If you choose wrongly you won't be able to stick to your diet.

Planning Healthy Foods

To maximize the benefits of the 16:8 diet, you should eat healthy foods as much as possible. If you fill up on foods that are rich in nutrients, you won't be hungry or crave unhealthy foods. This will help you to stick to your new way of eating in the long-term.

While you can enjoy some snacks and treats, you should balance every meal with a variety of wholefoods. Some of the best include:

- Fruits like bananas, apples, oranges, pears, peaches and berries
- Vegetables like tomatoes, leafy greens, cucumbers, cauliflower and broccoli
- Wholegrains like oats, rice, quinoa, buckwheat and barley
- Healthy fats like coconut oil, avocados and olive oil
- Lean protein like poultry, fish, seeds, nuts, eggs and legumes

If you binge on junk food, you could end up negating the benefits of this diet. Therefore, you should still keep unhealthy choices to a minimum.

Choosing Calorie-Free Beverages

You can drink any of your preferred beverages during your eating window. At least within reason! If you drink several family-sized bottles of full-fat soda you probably won't lose weight!

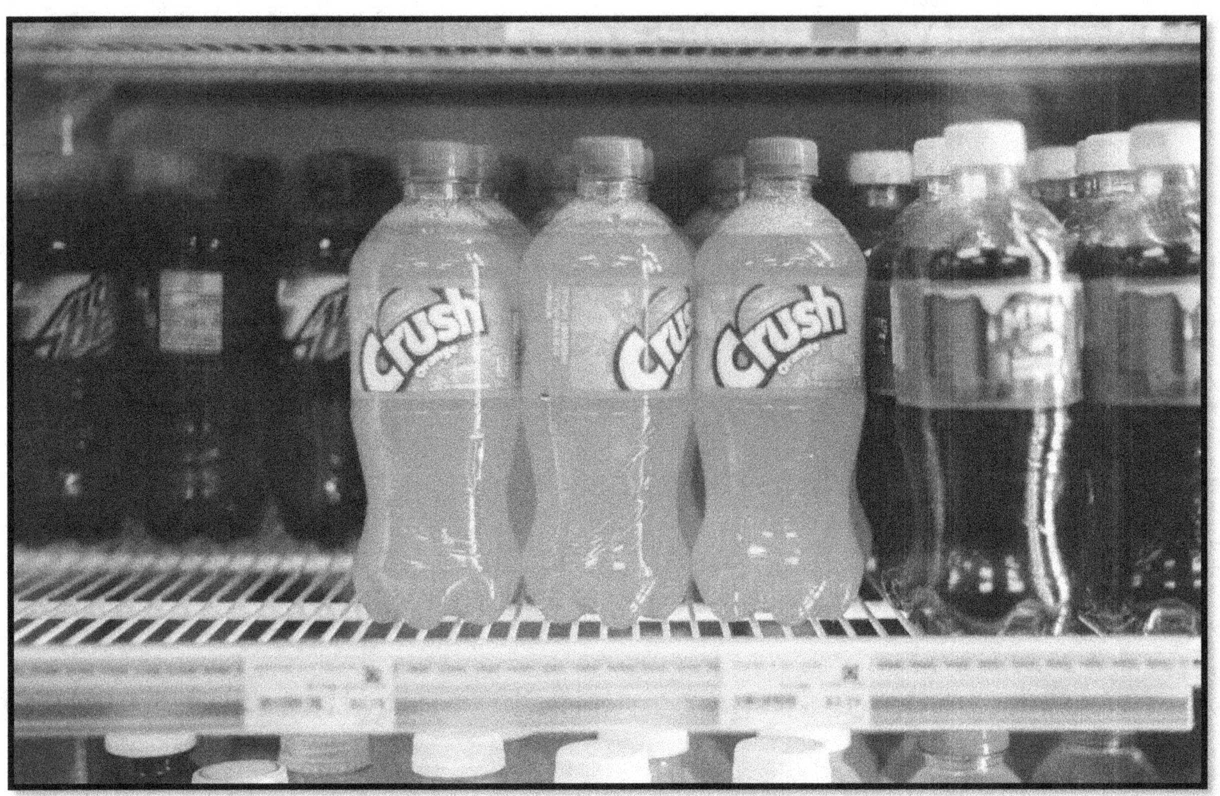

In your fasting window, you need to only consume calorie-free beverages. If you consume any beverage containing calories you are essentially breaking your fast. This spoils your entire eating regime.

Water, green tea, unsweetened coffee and tea without milk are all good choices. They will also help you to control your appetite and keep you hydrated until you break your fast.

A Weekly Timetable

Your weekly 16:8 eating timetable will vary depending on which eating window you choose. Here are three samples to suit different schedules:

Early Eating Meal Plan

Mon	Tues	Wed	Thurs	Fri	Sat	Sun
8 a.m. - breakfast	8 a.m. - breakfast	8 a.m. - breakfast	8 a.m. - breakfast	8 a.m. - breakfast	8 a.m. - breakfast	8 a.m. - breakfast
10 a.m. snack	10 a.m. snack	10 a.m. snack	10 a.m. snack	10 a.m. snack	10 a.m. snack	10 a.m. snack
12 noon - lunch	12 noon - lunch	12 noon - lunch	12 noon - lunch	12 noon - lunch	12 noon - lunch	12 noon – lunch
Evening – calorie-free beverages	Evening – calorie-free beverages	Evening – calorie-free beverages	Evening – calorie-free beverages	Evening – calorie-free beverages	Evening – calorie-free beverages	Evening – calorie-free beverages

Average Eating Meal Plan

Mon	Tues	Wed	Thurs	Fri	Sat	Sun
9 a.m. – calorie-free beverage	9 a.m. – calorie-free beverage	9 a.m. – calorie-free beverage	9 a.m. – calorie-free beverage	9 a.m. – calorie-free beverage	9 a.m. – calorie-free beverage	9 a.m. – calorie-free beverage
11 a.m. -	11 a.m. -	11 a.m. -	11 a.m. -	11 a.m. -	11 a.m. -	11 a.m. -

breakfast	breakfast	breakfast	breakfast	breakfast	breakfast	breakfast
2 p.m. lunch	2 p.m. lunch	2 p.m. lunch	2 p.m. lunch	2 p.m. lunch	2 p.m. lunch	2 p.m. lunch
4 p.m. snack	4 p.m. snack	4 p.m. snack	4 p.m. snack	4 p.m. snack	4 p.m. snack	4 p.m. snack
6 p.m. dinner	6 p.m. dinner	6 p.m. dinner	6 p.m. dinner	6 p.m. dinner	6 p.m. dinner	6 p.m. dinner

Late Eating Meal Plan

Mon	Tues	Wed	Thurs	Fri	Sat	Sun
11 a.m. – calorie-free beverage	11 a.m. – calorie-free beverage	11 a.m. – calorie-free beverage	11 a.m. – calorie-free beverage	11 a.m. – calorie-free beverage	11 a.m. – calorie-free beverage	11 a.m. – calorie-free beverage
1 p.m. snack	1 p.m. snack	1 p.m. snack	1 p.m. snack	1 p.m. snack	1 p.m. snack	1 p.m. snack
4 p.m. lunch	4 p.m. lunch	4 p.m. lunch	4 p.m. lunch	4 p.m. lunch	4 p.m. lunch	4 p.m. lunch
6 p.m. snack	6 p.m. snack	6 p.m. snack	6 p.m. snack	6 p.m. snack	6 p.m. snack	6 p.m. snack
9 p.m. dinner	9 p.m. dinner	9 p.m. dinner	9 p.m. dinner	9 p.m. dinner	9 p.m. dinner	9 p.m. dinner

6

A PROTOCOL FOR
24-HOUR
INTERMITTENT FASTING

Chapter 6 – A Protocol for 24-Hour Intermittent Fasting

If the 16:8 diet isn't right for you, you may want to consider 24-hour fasting. This is known as the Eat-Stop-Eat method. It involves one or two non-consecutive days of fasting every week.

Introduction to the Eat-Stop-Eat Method

This method was devised by Brad Pilon who wrote a book about this way of eating. His methodology was based on Canadian research into the effect of short-term fasts on metabolic health. The idea behind Pilon's method is to re-evaluate all you've learned about timing of meals and meal frequency.

This diet is quite easy to implement. You simply choose one day or two non-consecutive days of the week in which you won't eat for 24 hours. You can eat normally on the other five or six days. It's advisable, though, to eat healthily for the best results.

Although it sounds counterintuitive, you'll still be eating on every calendar day with this fast. How does this work?

Imagine you decide to fast from 9 a.m. on Monday until 9 a.m. on Tuesday. You eat your last meal on the Monday morning before 9 a.m. You can then eat your next meal on Tuesday morning after 9 a.m.

During your fasting hours, you should stay well-hydrated. Drink lots of water and other beverages with no calories like unsweetened, milk-free tea or coffee.

Choosing Your Fasting Days

If you want to try the Eat-Stop-Eat method, you'll need to choose the right fasting days for you. This will be down to individual choice. First, you'll need to choose whether to fast for one day or two. You'll probably find it easier to start out with one fasting day per week. When you're used to it, you can increase it to two days weekly. Don't exceed that number of days though.

Some people find it easier to fast at the weekend because they don't have to focus at work. Others would prefer to fast on workdays so they have distractions to stop them thinking about food. You will need to determine your own preferences.

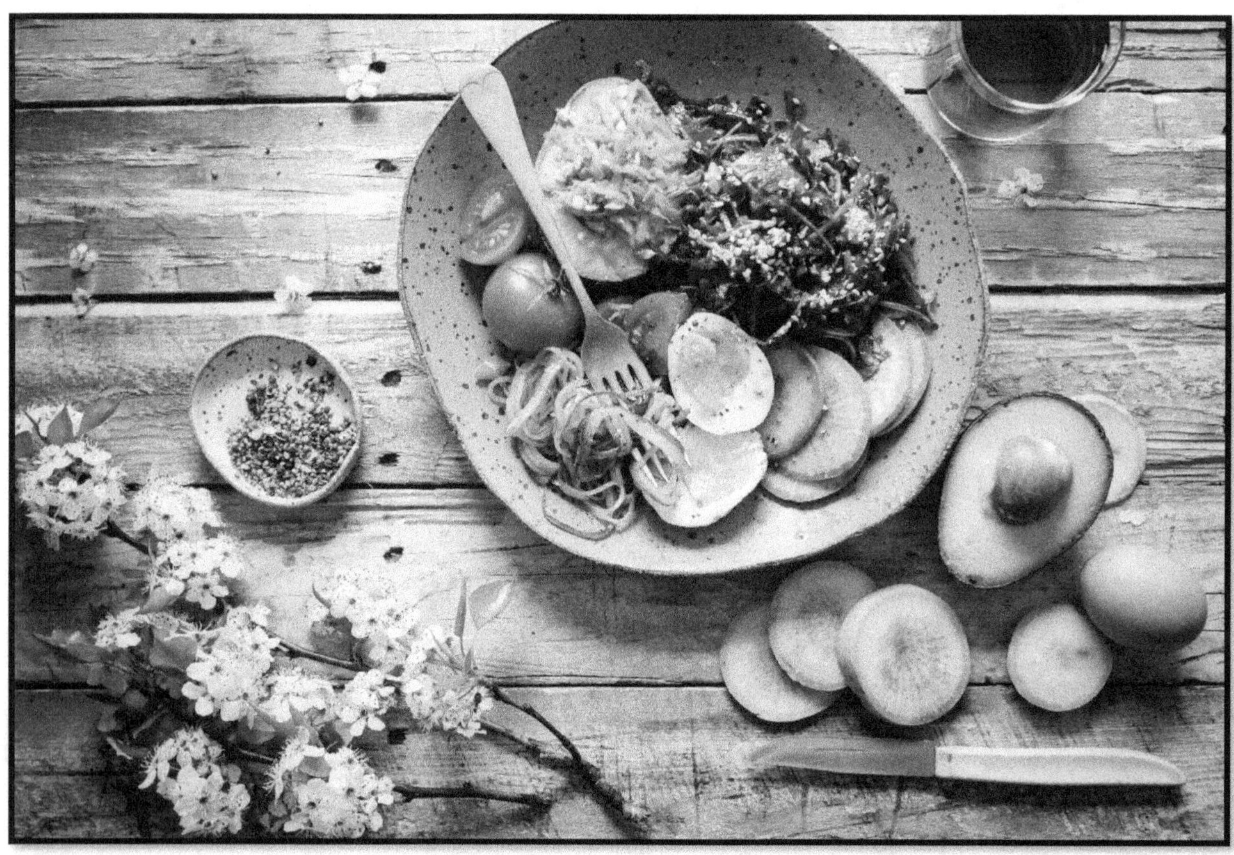

Remember, though, if you choose to do two days of fasting, they cannot be consecutive. This would be too long an extended period of fasting. You may wish to space your two fast days out fairly evenly. Alternatively, you may wish to space them just a day apart then enjoy eating the rest of the week. You may need to experiment to find the right pattern for you.

A Weekly Timetable

These are some sample timetables to help you plan your 24-hour fasts:

One Day Fast Meal Plan

Mon-Tues	Tues-Weds	Weds-Thurs	Thurs-Fri	Fri-Sat	Sat-Sun	Sun-Mon
9 a.m. – 9 a.m. eat normally	9 a.m.- 9 a.m. fast	9 a.m. – 9 a.m. eat normally	9 a.m. – 9 a.m. eat normally	9 a.m. - 9 a.m. eat normally	9 a.m. - 9 a.m. eat normally	9 a.m. – 9 a.m. eat normally

Two Day Fast Meal Plan

Mon-Tues	Tues-Weds	Weds-Thurs	Thurs-Fri	Fri-Sat	Sat-Sun	Sun-Mon
9 a.m. – 9 a.m. eat normally	9 a.m.- 9 a.m. fast	9 a.m. – 9 a.m. eat normally	9 a.m. – 9 a.m. fast	9 a.m. – 9 a.m. eat normally	9 a.m. – 9 a.m. eat normally	9 a.m. – 9 a.m. eat normally

You may prefer to begin your fast period at an earlier or later hour of the day. We have suggested 9 a.m. – 9 a.m. on the next day. However, you may prefer 7 a.m.- 7 a.m., or even 12 noon to 12 noon. You need to choose the right times for you as well as the right days.

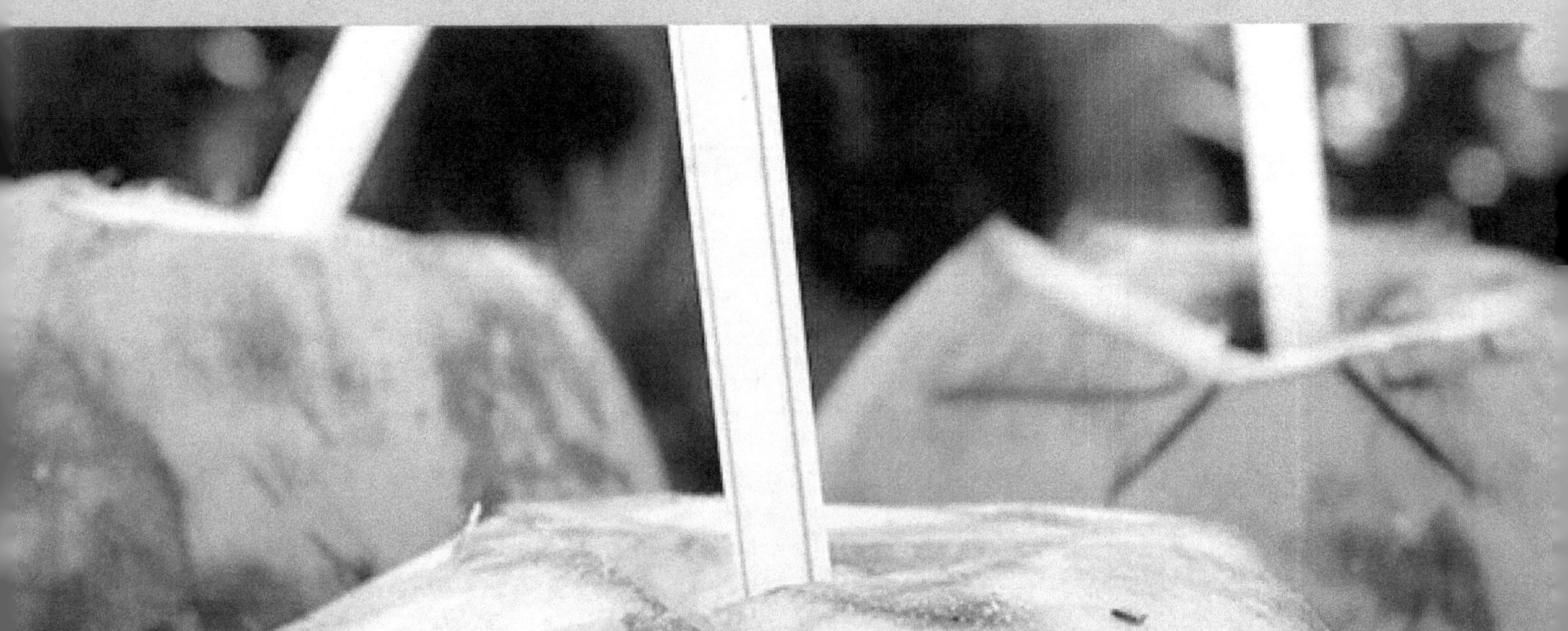

Chapter 7 – Other Types of Intermittent Fasting

Although 24-hour and 16:8 intermittent fasting are the two most popular types, there are several others. Here, we'll take a closer look at five other kinds of fasting regimes that several people follow.

20:4 Fasting

20:4 fasting is sometimes called the Warrior Diet. It was one of the earliest diets to involve intermittent fasting. Made popular by Ori Hofmekler, a fitness expert, this diet involves eating one large meal in the evening. This large meal takes place in a four-hour eating window.

During the other 20 hours of the day, only small amounts of raw vegetables and fruits can be eaten. The food choices for this diet should be healthy – similar to those on the Paleo diet. They should be unprocessed wholefoods that contain no artificial ingredients.

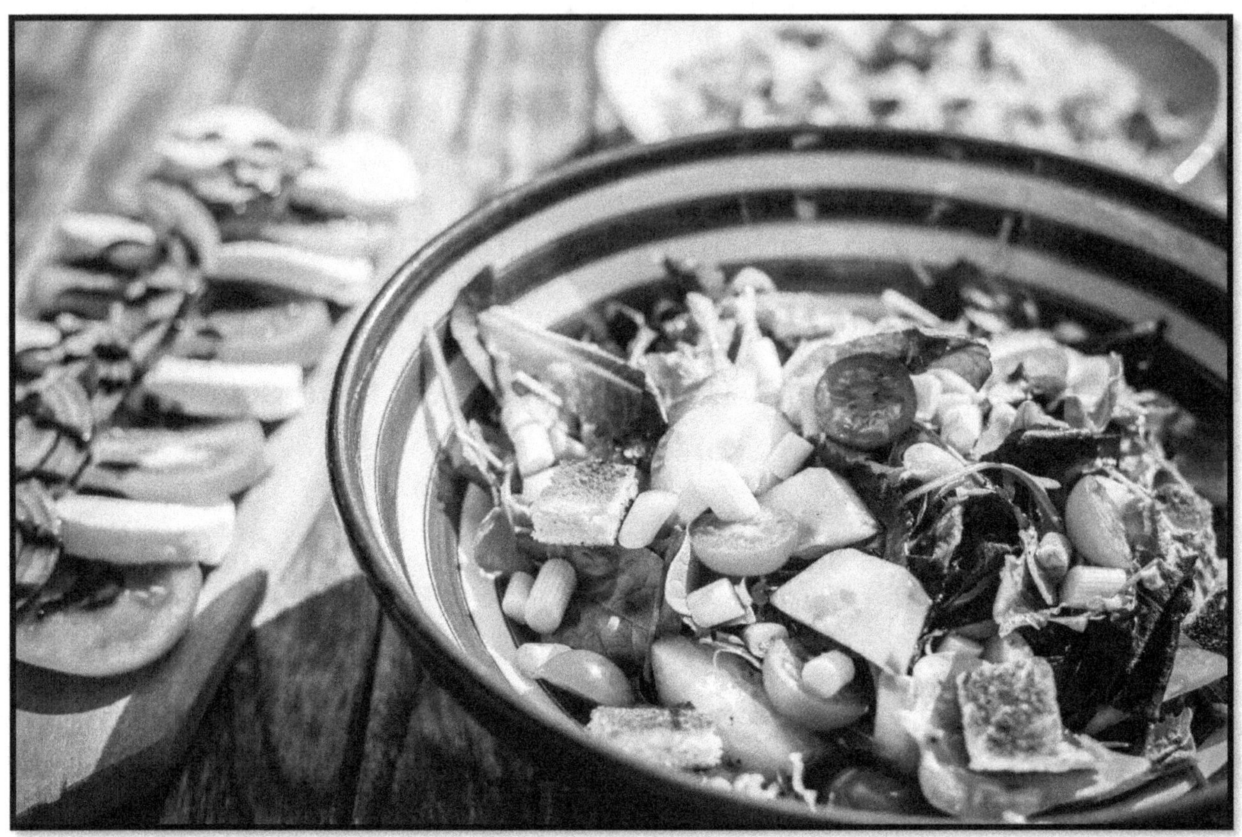

A timetable for this diet looks like this:

Mon	Tues	Wed	Thurs	Fri	Sat	Sun
Midnight – 4 p.m. – small amounts of fruit and vegetables	Midnight – 4 p.m. – small amounts of fruit and vegetables	Midnight – 4 p.m. – small amounts of fruit and vegetables	Midnight – 4 p.m. – small amounts of fruit and vegetables	Midnight – 4 p.m. – small amounts of fruit and vegetables	Midnight – 4 p.m. – small amounts of fruit and vegetables	Midnight – 4 p.m. – small amounts of fruit and vegetables
4 p.m.- 8 p.m. – Large Meal	4 p.m. - 8 p.m. – Large Meal	4 p.m. - 8 p.m. – Large Meal	4 p.m. - 8 p.m. – Large Meal	4 p.m. - 8 p.m. – Large Meal	4 p.m. - 8 p.m. – Large Meal	4 p.m. - 8 p.m. – Large Meal
8 p.m. - midnight - fast	8 p.m. - midnight – fast	8 p.m. - midnight – fast	8 p.m. - midnight – fast	8 p.m. - midnight – fast	8 p.m. - midnight – fast	8 p.m. - midnight - fast

5:2 Fasting

This popular form of intermittent fasting involves eating normally for five days every week. The remaining two days, calories should be restricted to 500 – 600. Sometimes called the Fast Diet, this way of eating was made popular by Michael Mosley, a journalist. Women are recommended to eat 500 calories on their fasting days. Men can have 600 calories on their fast days.

You can choose which two days you prefer to fast. However, it's best if they aren't consecutive. On those days, you can choose to eat one meal or two small meals. Many people prefer to eat two meals of 250/300 calories each.

This is a sample timetable for this way of eating:

Mon	Tues	Weds	Thurs	Fri	Sat	Sun
Eat normally	Eat 500/600 calories	Eat normally	Eat normally	Eat 500/600 calories	Eat normally	Eat normally

36-Hour Fasting

The 36-hour fast plan means you'll be fasting for a full day. Unlike the Eat-Stop-Eat method, you won't be eating something every calendar day.

If, for example, you finish dinner at 7 p.m. on day one, you skip all your meals on day two. You won't eat your next meal until day 3 at 7 a.m. This equals a 36-hour fast.

There is some evidence to suggest this kind of fasting period can produce a quicker result. It may also be beneficial for diabetics. It may also be more problematic though since you'll be going for extended periods without food.

A timetable for this eating plan looks like this:

Mon	Tues	Weds	Thurs	Fri	Sat	Sun
Midnight - 7 a.m. Eat normally	Midnight - 7 a.m. Fast	Midnight – 7 a.m. Fast	Midnight - 7 a.m. Eat normally	Midnight - 7 a.m. Eat normally	Midnight - 7 a.m. Eat normally	Midnight - 7 a.m. Eat normally
7 a.m. – 7 p.m. Eat normally	7 a.m. – 7 p.m. Fast	7 a.m. – 7 p.m. Eat normally	7 a.m. – 7 p.m. Eat normally	7 a.m. – 7 p.m. Eat normally	7 a.m. – 7 p.m. Eat normally	7 a.m. – 7 p.m. Eat normally
7 p.m. – midnight Fast	7 p.m. – midnight Fast	7 p.m. – midnight Eat normally	7 p.m. – midnight Eat normally	7 p.m. – midnight Eat normally	7 p.m. – midnight Eat normally	7 p m – midnight Eat normally

Alternate Day Fasting

This way of fasting means that you fast for a full 24 hours every alternate day. Some versions of this IF diet allow you to eat up to 500 calories on a fast day. Others only allow you to have calorie-free beverages.

This isn't the best option for any newcomers to intermittent fasting. You go to bed feeling hungry several nights each week. This is hard to maintain in the long-term.

A timetable for this way of eating looks like this:

Mon	Tues	Weds	Thurs	Fri	Sat	Sun
midnight-midnight	Midnight-midnight	Midnight – midnight	Midnight – midnight	Midnight – Midnight	Midnight – Midnight	Midnight – midnight
Eat normally	Fast	Eat Normally	Fast	Eat normally	Fast	Eat normally

Extended Fasts

Following the 16:8 or Eat-Stop-Eat method is quite simple. Some people, though, are keen to push the benefits of intermittent fasting to the limit. They prefer to do a 42-hour fast.

This involves eating dinner on day 1, say at 6 p.m. All meals would be skipped on the next day. On day 3, you would then eat your breakfast at noon. This would be a total fasting time of 42 hours.

If you try this way of eating, you shouldn't restrict your calorie intake during your eating window.

It's technically possible to extend fasts for longer periods of time. In fact, the world record stands at 382 days. Of course, that isn't recommended!

Some people do try 7 to 14 day fasts due to the theoretical benefits they are said to provide. Some people say that a seven-day fast can help prevent cancer. Others say that longer fasts promote mental clarity. These benefits are unproven and are theoretical. It's probably best, therefore, to stick to one of the tried and tested IF plans outlined above.

CHAPTER 8

HOW TO MAXIMIZE YOUR INTERMITTENT FASTING RESULTS

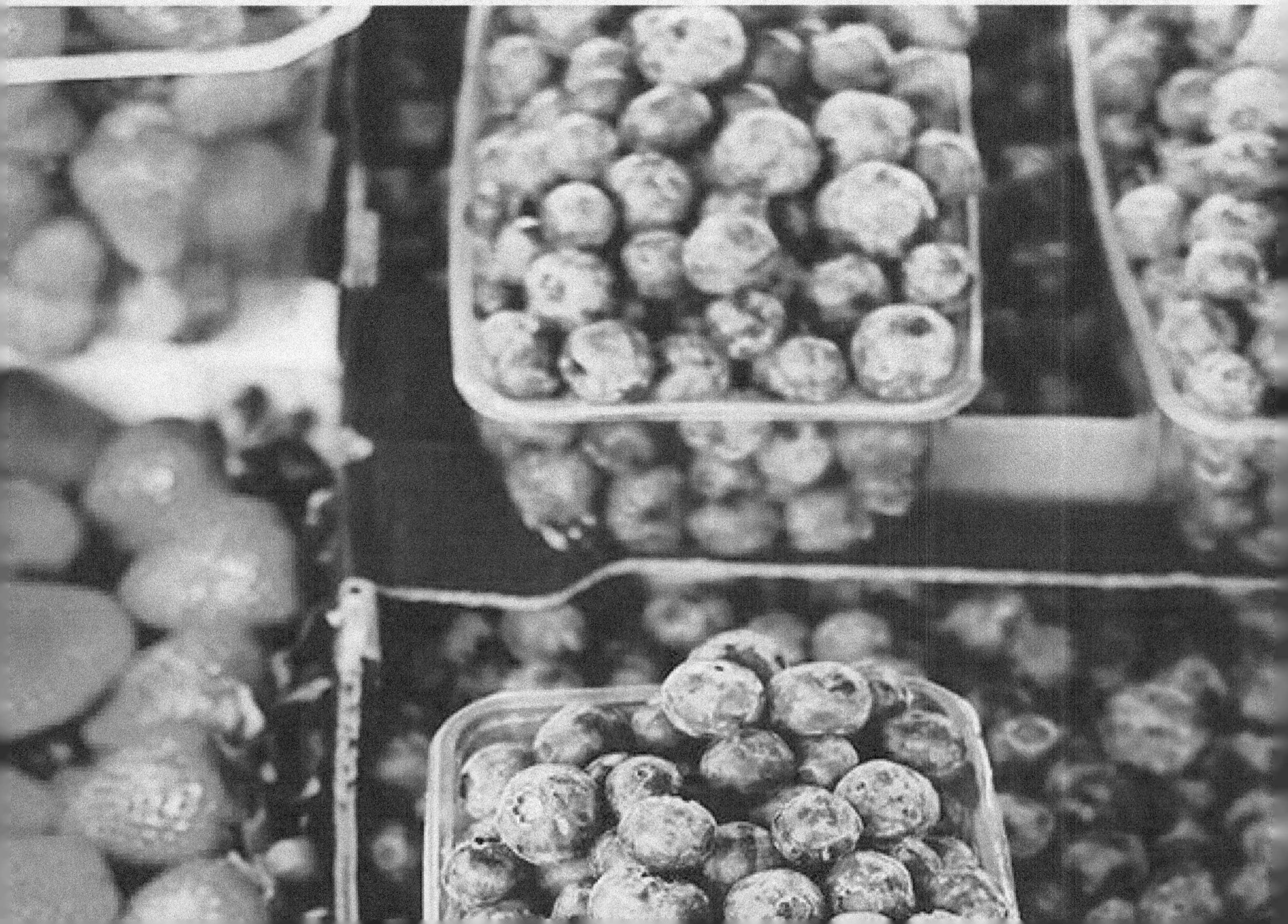

Chapter 8 – How to Maximize Your Intermittent Fasting Results

Are you ready to try intermittent fasting? Whether you're doing it for weight loss or for the other benefits, you will probably want to maximize your results.

Luckily, there are a few things you can do to get as much benefit as possible from your eating regime. Here, we take a look at some things you can try to speed your weight loss.

Exercise and Intermittent Fasting

There is some research to show that if you exercise while fasting, there are additional benefits. There is an impact on your metabolism and muscle biochemistry. This is linked to your insulin sensitivity and blood sugar level. If you exercise while fasting, your glycogen (or stored carbs) are depleted. This means you'll burn more fat.

To get the best result, eat protein following your workout. This will build and maintain your muscles. It will also promote better recovery. You should also follow up strength training with carbs within a half hour of your workout.

It's wise to eat food close to any modern or high-intensity exercise session. You should also drink a lot more water to stay well-hydrated. Keeping up your electrolyte level is important. Coconut water can be useful for this.

You may feel a little lightheaded or dizzy if you work out while fasting. If you experience this, take a break. It's important to listen to your body. If you're doing a longer fast, you may find gentle exercise like pilates, yoga or walking are better. They will help to burn fat without making you feel unwell.

Choosing the Right Regime for You

To maximize the results of your intermittent fasting, you'll need to choose the right regime. As you've seen there are several different types of intermittent fasting diet. Not all are suitable for everyone. You need to find one that works well for your lifestyle and that makes your life easier.

When you choose the right regime, you'll stick to it in the long-term. So, here are some questions to ask yourself to help you choose wisely.

Are you already eating healthily?

Fasting is harder if you're currently eating a standard American diet. This is because it is high carb, full of sugars and very addictive. If you jump straight into extreme fasting, you'll experience symptoms of withdrawal from sugar. This makes it hard to stick to your new diet.

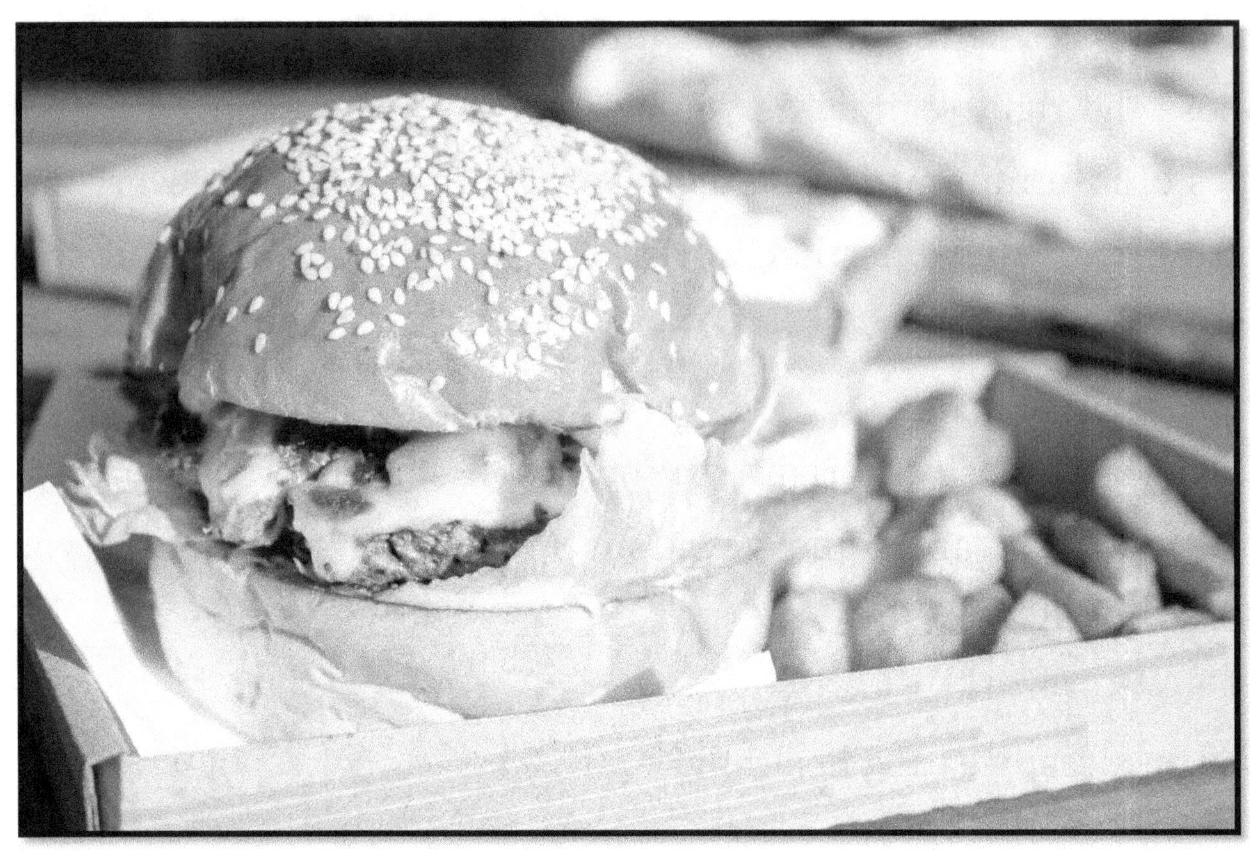

If you usually eat processed foods regularly, try beginning with a short fasting window. Meanwhile, detox from sugar and begin to eat more cleanly. Stop snacking and introduce wholefoods into your diet. You can then increase the fasting window if necessary. On the other hand, if you already eat healthily, you can start with a longer fast window.

Can you manage to go for long periods without eating?

Some people are able to manage fasting for a whole day. Others can only manage a few hours. You may need to experiment. Focus on the way fasting makes you feel. If you struggle to fast for long periods, choose a method like the 5:2 or 16:8. If you find it easy, you may be able to opt for a 36-hour fast straight away.

How does your schedule look?

It's easier to fast if you're busy and distracted from thinking about food. If you fast at work or while you're working on something, you'll probably feel less hungry. If you work out, you may want to end your fasting window straight after exercising.

If you answer these questions, you'll be best-placed to choose the right regime to suit your life and preferences. This will give you the best chance of success.

Adding in Keto

Some experts say that if you combine intermittent fasting with the keto diet, you'll lose more weight. So, what does this involve?

The keto (or ketogenic) diet is a specific way of eating in which most calories come from healthy fats. The remaining calories are derived from protein. Very few, if any, carbohydrates are consumed on this diet.

This low-carb, high-fat diet encourages your body to burn fat, not sugars, to produce energy. If your body lacks sufficient carbs to carry out everyday activities, fat is broken down by the liver. It produces ketones and they are then used as a fuel for energy. The process is known as ketosis. Hence the name "keto".

Like intermittent fasting, keto diets have a number of benefits. They can boost weight loss, reduce your blood sugar level and improve your brain function. Many people say it helps to reduce problems like diabetes and obesity.

If you combine keto dieting with IF, the amount of time you're in ketosis increases. This could make you feel more energetic, less hungry and speed your weight loss.

CHAPTER 9

HOW TO GET STARTED WITH INTERMITTENT FASTING

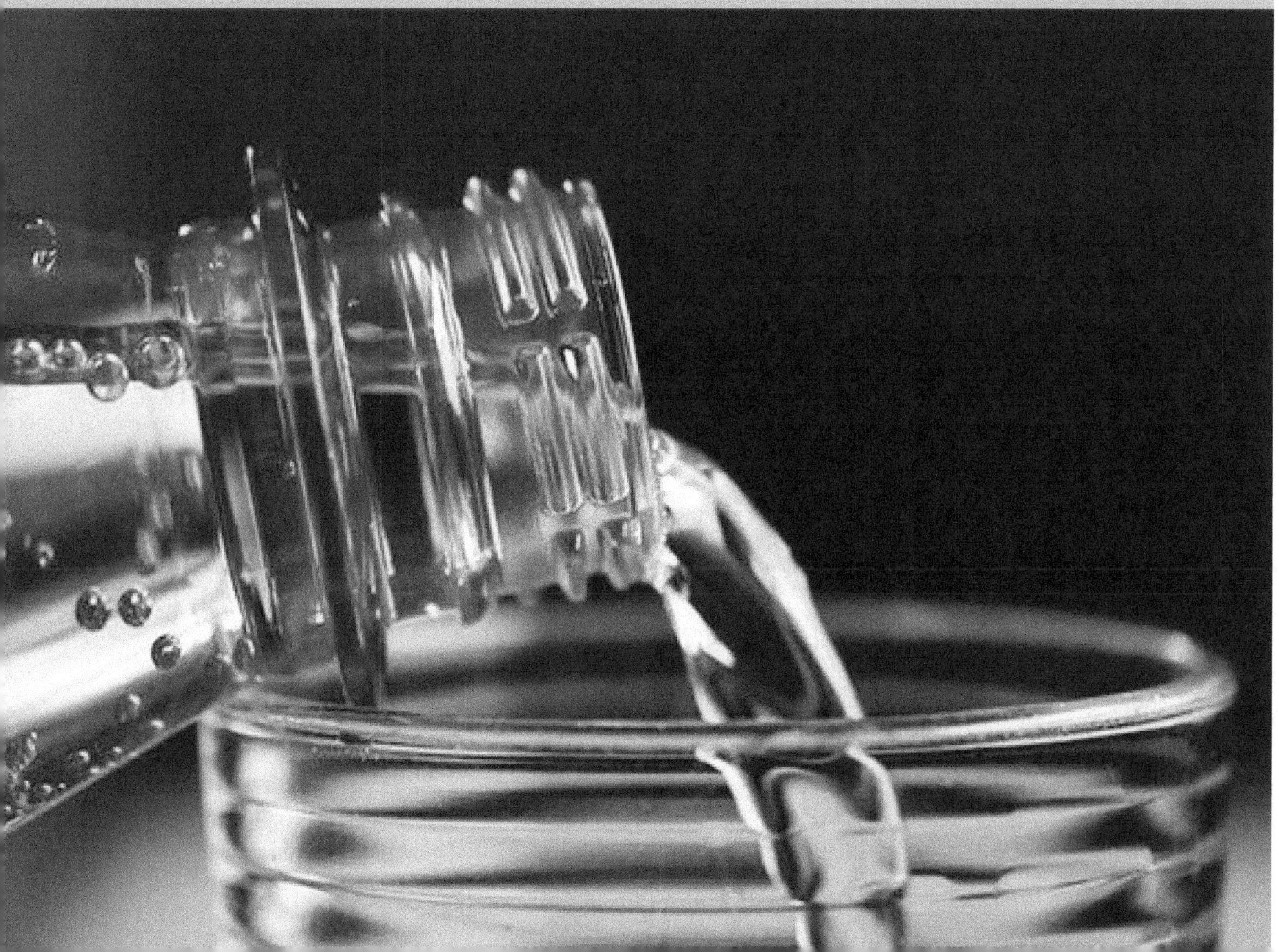

Chapter 9 – How to get Started with Intermittent Fasting

If you're convinced of the benefits of intermittent fasting, you'll need to know how to get started. After all, embarking on any new regime can be complicated. So, how can you get yourself off to the best possible start? Here are some top tips.

Starting with a less Rigorous Regime

It may be tempting to try to lose as much weight as possible by starting out with a long fast. However, bear in mind this may not be the best approach. As we've already mentioned, it can be difficult to fast for extended periods if you've never done it before. If you're used to a high-carb, high-sugar, processed foods diet, you'll struggle to fast for 36 hours straight off.

If you find your first fast impossibly hard, you'll probably put off the whole idea. Even if you aren't, the likelihood of sticking to it for any length of time is low.

It's recommended to try any intermittent fasting plan for at least a month. This will give you enough time to see whether it's working for you or not. It will be very difficult for someone inexperienced to stick to an extended fast regime in the long-term.

It's therefore best to opt for one of the less rigorous regimes to start with. The 5:2 diet allows you to eat some food every day. In fact, you can eat your regular meals on five days of the week. The other two, you still get 500 or 600 calories to play with. This should give you plenty of options as long as you make healthy choices. Choose your meals wisely, and you'll experience the benefits without ever feeling hungry.

Alternatively, try the popular 16:8 method. For a large proportion of your fasting time you'll be asleep. You'll then be free to eat whatever you like (within reason) during your 8-hour eating window. Many people like the freedom that this offers. When they get used to the 16-hour fast, they find this way of eating quite simple.

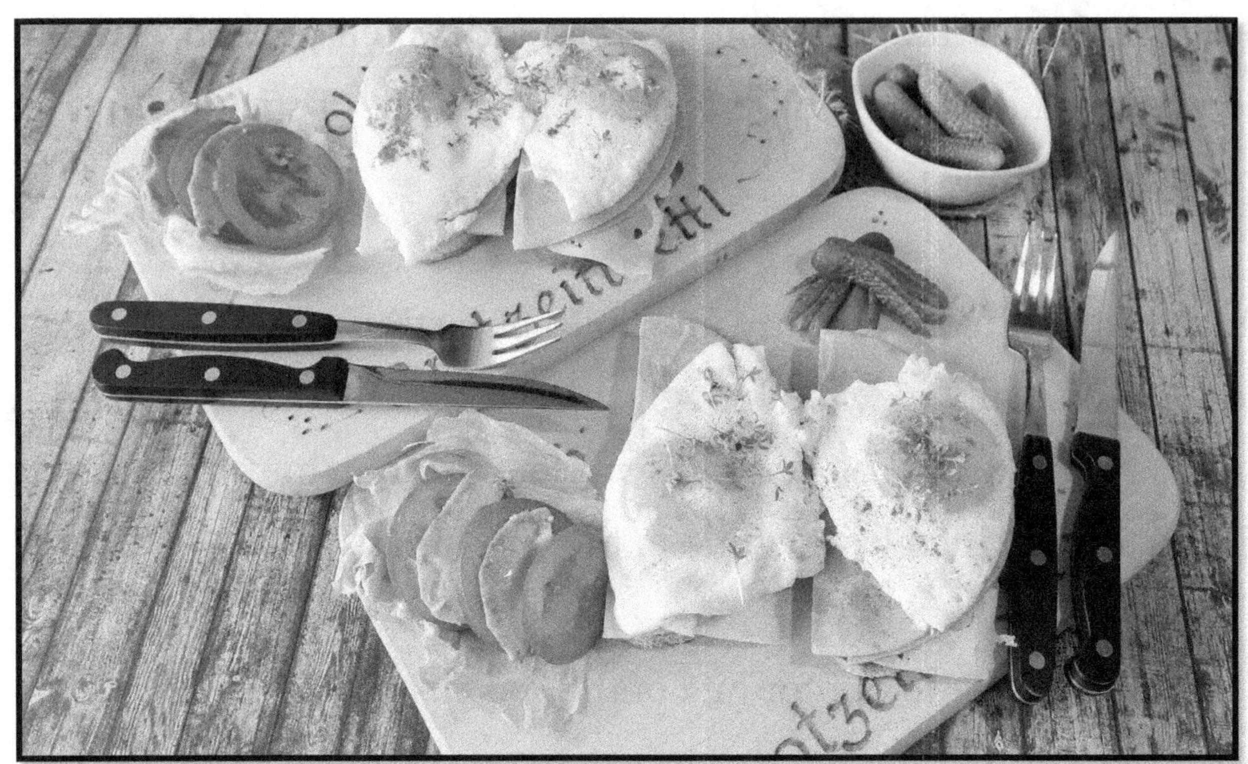

If you want to work up to longer fasts once you're used to fasting, you can. However, many people continue to follow their initial plan in the long-term and experience good results.

Staying Hydrated

Whatever type of intermittent fasting plan you try, you need to stay well-hydrated. Fasting is only referring to food and calorie-containing beverages. It doesn't mean you can't have water and other calorie-free drinks. In fact, you should drink more of them!

Staying hydrated will ensure that toxins can be flushed effectively from your body. This will help to promote your weight loss and wellness goals. It will also help you to stay healthy in other ways. Your skin will be healthier. Your bowel habits will be more regular. You'll also avoid headaches and other problems associated with dehydration.

Drinking calorie-free beverages during your fasting window can also help to prevent you from feeling hungry. Often, we think we're hungry, but we're actually thirsty instead. If you drink a glass of water when you're beginning to feel hungry, you'll continue fasting for longer.

Try Experimenting with Different Eating Patterns

We have suggested some eating plan timetables above, however that doesn't mean you need to stick to them. The days and times that we have suggested are just examples. They may not work for you. You need to choose the right days and eating patterns to fit your lifestyle, preferences and needs.

Perhaps you prefer to begin eating as soon as you get up and then have your last meal early. Or maybe breaking your fast in the early afternoon and having a last meal just before bed is best.

You may prefer to fast at the weekend so you don't need to worry about feeling tired at work. Or fasting on a weekday may be right for you so you have distractions.

There is no single perfect IF plan for everyone. That means you may need to do a little experimentation. Weigh up the pros and cons of all the regimes that we've suggested. Think about which one you're most drawn to and give it a try. It's best to try to give it a month to see how well it works for you. If you're having problems, it's time to go back to the drawing board. Try a different intermittent fasting regime to see if that better suits your lifestyle. Or move your eating windows around a little to see if it becomes more manageable.

Don't be afraid to experiment – after all, experimentation could be the key to success.

10

ADDRESSING COMMON QUESTIONS

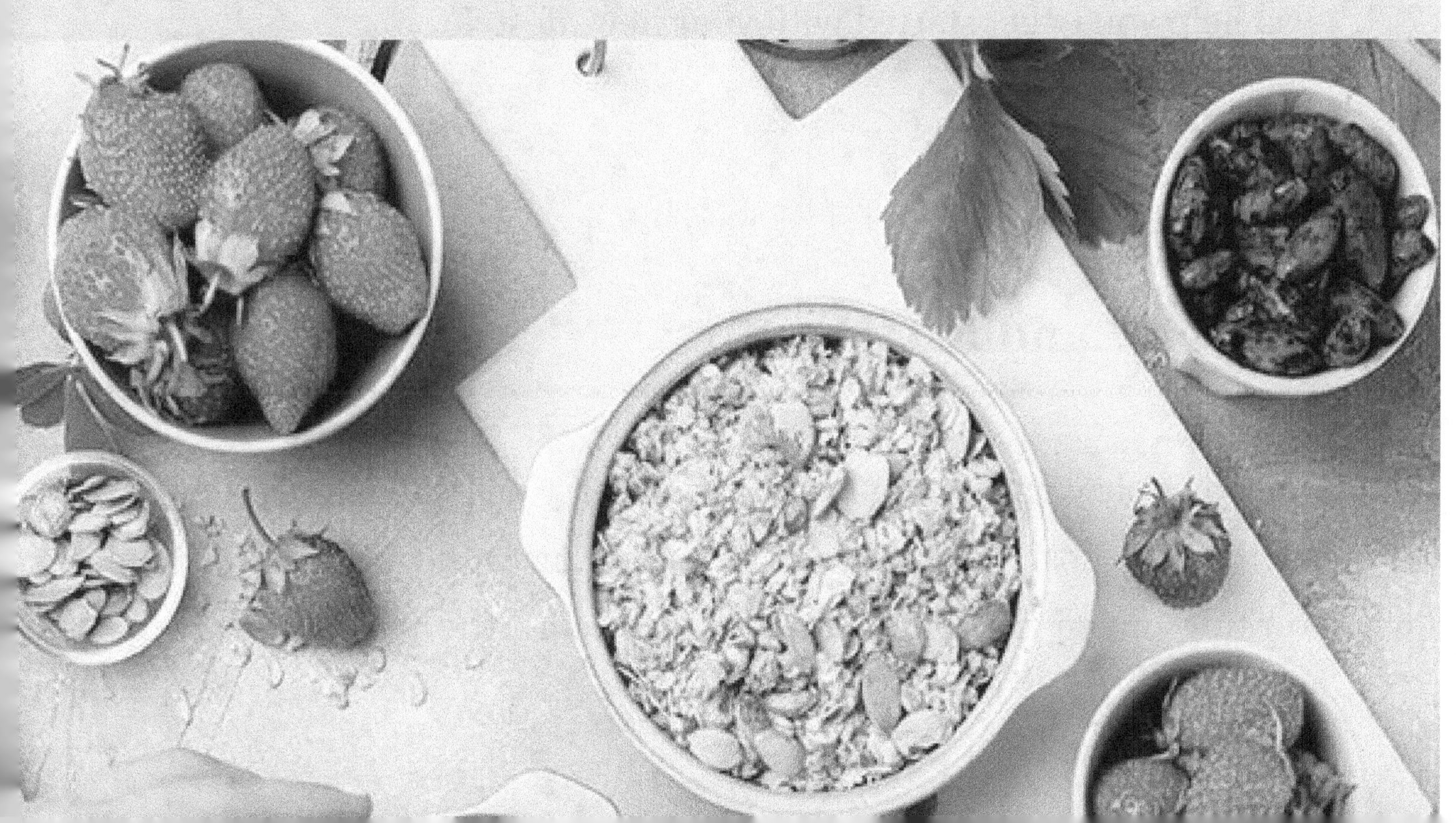

Chapter 10 – Addressing Common Questions

When you're keen to start intermittent fasting, you'll want all the information you need at your fingertips. Although we've addressed all the key points in the first nine chapters, there are a few more questions to answer.

Here, we address some of the most common questions about intermittent fasting. Hopefully, the answers will help you to make a final decision about whether IF could be right for you. It should also help you to get started with your new lifestyle.

Exercise and Fasting

Many people wonder whether they can carry on exercising if they're fasting. In most cases, intermittent fasting won't stop you from working out in the long-run. It may take a little time, though, to adjust to your new regime. Some people who follow this lifestyle even find they're more energetic while fasting!

Some people worry that they'll lose muscle if they fast. This is something that is a danger with any diet. However, you can avoid this happening. If you eat plenty of protein in your eating window and do regular resistance training you should be fine.

It's advisable to exercise at the end of your fasting period. Usually, you'll feel hungry around 30 minutes after finishing your work out. If you break your fast at that time, you'll feel satisfied.

What Should you eat During your Eating Window?

When you follow an IF lifestyle, there are no restrictions about what you can eat in your eating window. This is why it is so different from other ways of dieting. You aren't restricted to amounts or specific food types. However, it's wise to remember that you should still make healthy choices. If you over-indulge regularly you won't see the benefits of IF.

The best solution is to eat a balanced diet in your eating window. This will help you to maintain your energy level while still losing weight. Foods that are dense in nutrients like seeds, beans, nuts, wholegrains, vegetables and fruits are good choices. You should also consume plenty of lean protein.

There are certain foods that are especially beneficial if you follow this way of eating:

- Avocados – yes, they're high in calorie. However, they are packed with monounsaturated fats. This makes them very satiating. If you add a half avocado to your meal you'll feel much fuller.
- Fish – you should try to eat a minimum of 8 ounces of fish every week. Fish is packed with protein, healthy fats and vitamin D. It's also good for your brain health.
- Cruciferous vegetables – foods such as cauliflower, Brussels sprouts and broccoli are good choices. They're packed with fiber to help you avoid constipation and feel more full.
- Potatoes – many people worry that potatoes are bad for you. However, they're very satisfying and will keep you full for longer.

- Legumes and beans – although these are carbs, they're low calorie and give you lots of energy. They are also packed with protein and fiber.
- Probiotics – eating foods rich in probiotics like sauerkraut, kefir and kombucha helps keep your gut happy. This will help you to avoid stomach issues when you're adjusting to this diet.
- Berries – strawberries, blueberries and others are packed with nutrients like vitamin C. They're also rich in flavonoids – something that is known to boost weight loss.
- Eggs – every egg has a massive 6 grams of protein. Simple and quick to cook, eggs make you feel full.
- Nuts – yes, nuts are high in calories. However, they're packed with polyunsaturated fat that helps you feel full.
- Wholegrains – yes, wholegrains are also carbs! However, they're full of protein and fiber. You don't need to eat too much to feel full for longer. A study has even shown that eating wholegrains can boost your metabolism.

What can you Have in Your Fasting Period?

So, you know what you can eat in your eating window. What can you have in your fasting period? The answer depends on which fast you're doing.

If you're doing the 5:2 diet, you can eat up to 500 or 600 calories on your fast days. Obviously, that's quite restrictive. So, you can maximize the amount you can eat by including lots of low calorie, high-nutrient foods. Vegetables and fruits are staples of your fast days.

If you're doing any of the other fasting methods, you can't eat any solid foods at all. You also can't have any drinks that contain calories. Luckily, though, there are lots of beverages you can have to stay hydrated.

It's obvious that you should have lots of water in your fasting window. Sparkling and still water are both fine. If you wish, you can add a squeeze of lime or lemon for a little more flavor. You could also add more flavor with some orange or cucumber slices. You can't add any artificially-sweetened enhancers though. These could damage your fast.

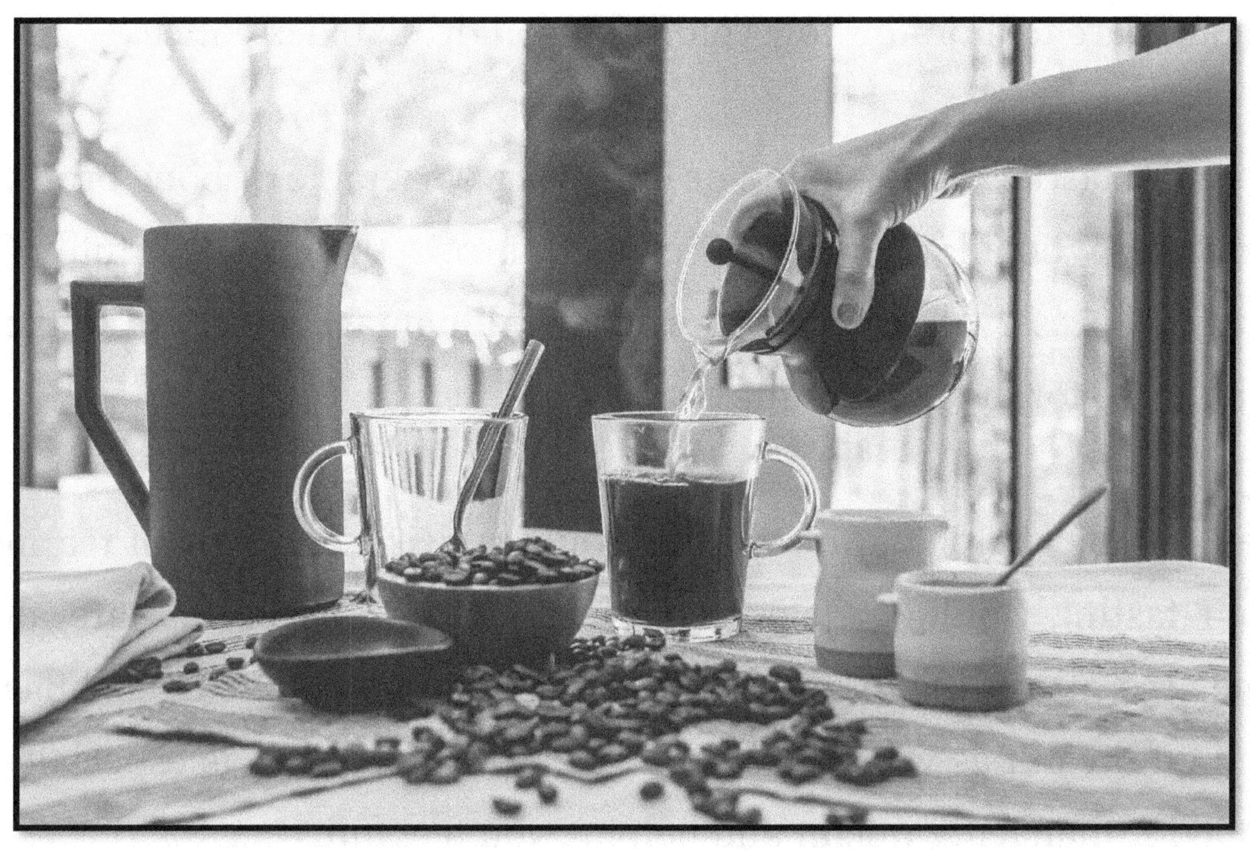

Another good beverage for your fasting period is black coffee. It contains no calories and won't affect your insulin levels. You can have decaffeinated or regular coffee but don't add milk or sweeteners. If you want more flavor, try adding cinnamon or other spices. Some people say that black coffee could enhance IF's benefits.

Caffeine may support the production of ketones. It can also help to support a healthy level of blood sugars in the long-run. A note of warning, though. Some people find that if they drink coffee during their fast they get an upset stomach or racing heart. You may need to take care to monitor how you feel if you drink black coffee.

If you're fasting for 24-hours or longer, try vegetable or bone broth. Don't use bouillon cubes or canned broth though. It's full of artificial preservatives and flavors that will damage your fast. Make it at home for the best results.

Tea can also help you to feel full. You can drink any type of tea in your fasting window. Oolong, black, green and herbal tea are all fine. Tea also helps to improve your fasting by supporting cellular and gut health as well as probiotic balance. Green tea is especially good for managing weight and helping you feel full.

Apple cider vinegar offers many health benefits. You can add this to the list of things you can have during your fasting period. It will support your blood sugar level and digestion. It could even boost the results of your fasting.

There are, however, some drinks that you need to avoid while you're fasting. You may not realize that "zero-calorie" sodas can break your fast. While diet sodas technically have no calories, they've been shown to inhibit fasting's positive effects. This is because they get their sweet flavor from aspartame or other artificial sweeteners. These trigger your insulin response. You should therefore avoid drinking them in your fast window.

Many people ask whether they can have coconut water or almond milk in their fast period. While both of these are healthy options with benefits for your wellness, they contain lots of sugar. Since sugar is a carbohydrate, you'll no longer be fasting if you consume it. You shouldn't drink these beverages in your fasting period.

One very common question is whether it's possible to drink alcohol if you're doing an IF diet. It's important to limit your consumption of alcohol to your eating window. This is because most alcoholic drinks contain a lot of calories and sugar. Therefore, drinking them will break your fast. Also, alcohol will have more effect on you if you have an empty stomach. Even a single glass of wine may make you feel unwell!

Can Children try Intermittent Fasting?

There is no specific evidence to say whether it's safe for children to try intermittent fasting or not. Some experts say that it's perfectly fine, especially for those who are already overweight. Others say it's a bad idea since children are going through a period of rapid growth. They need sufficient calories to support their development and growth. Children need to eat enough protein, vitamins and minerals. If they don't get enough, they could become ill. It's probably wise to speak to a doctor before putting a child on an IF diet.

Is Fasting Unhealthy?

It's only natural for people to ask whether fasting is unhealthy. Those who extol the virtues of more traditional diets say that fasting could slow your metabolism. This could cause you to put on weight, not lose it. Therefore, they say, fasting is unhealthy.

However, this isn't the case at all. People have been fasting for centuries with no ill effects. Studies carried out on people during Ramadan have shown that extended fasting causes no health issues for most people.

There are a few issues to bear in mind, though. Fasting isn't for everyone. Some people find it difficult to fit it into their lives. They struggle to sustain this lifestyle for extended periods. They may find it difficult to fit in socializing, work and exercise around fasting windows. This can lead to an inconsistent eating schedule that may have unhealthy consequences.

There are a few other issues to consider too. Some people who try IF begin to lose touch with the signals that tell them that they're full and hungry. This can make it hard to stick to IF in the long-run without developing an eating disorder.

Some people who are prone to eating disorders become obsessed with food and eating. Some binge during their eating window. Others push their fasting further and further and become fixated with not eating. It's therefore important to approach IF with caution if you have a history of disordered eating.

On the whole, though, IF isn't just not unhealthy, it can be positively good for you. It can help you to effectively manage your weight and avoid obesity. It can improve your metabolism and your insulin resistance. It can also decrease your inflammation and boost your cell repair as well as support a healthier gastrointestinal tract.

Conclusion

Now you know the benefits and possible problems associated with intermittent fasting. If you're ready to try it yourself, this book should tell you everything you need to know to get started.

Identify why you want to try intermittent fasting. You may want to lose weight or improve your health. You may just want to see if it makes you feel more focused and energetic. If you know which benefits you'd like to see, you'll be in a better position for success. You'll also be able to prioritize the strategy and foods that will be best for your goals.

As you've seen in this book, there are several different IF plans to choose from. You'll need to consider which one is right for you. You may prefer a daily approach with something like the 16:8 diet. Alternatively, a weekly plan like alternate day fasting or 5:2 may suit you best.

You'll need to consider your schedule and your personal preferences. Think about the times you get up and go to bed. When do you tend to get hungry? How busy are you during your day? Do you work out? The answers to these questions will help you choose your eating window.

If intermittent fasting is going to be successful for you, it needs to work effectively around your lifestyle. You need to be sure that you can keep up your diet in the long-term. You'll only be able to do that if it fits in with your needs. Remember that intermittent fasting should make your life easier, not harder. If it's too difficult to follow, you'll give up too quickly. You should try to follow the diet for a minimum of a month to see if it's working for you.

When you get intermittent fasting right, you should reap the benefits quickly. Not only should you lose weight, you should feel more energetic and healthy. You'll feel more focused and experience a wealth of health and wellness benefits. From a reduced chance of developing diabetes to a potentially longer lifespan, the advantages are numerous.

So, what are you waiting for? It's time to give intermittent fasting a try for yourself. You're sure to experience the benefits!